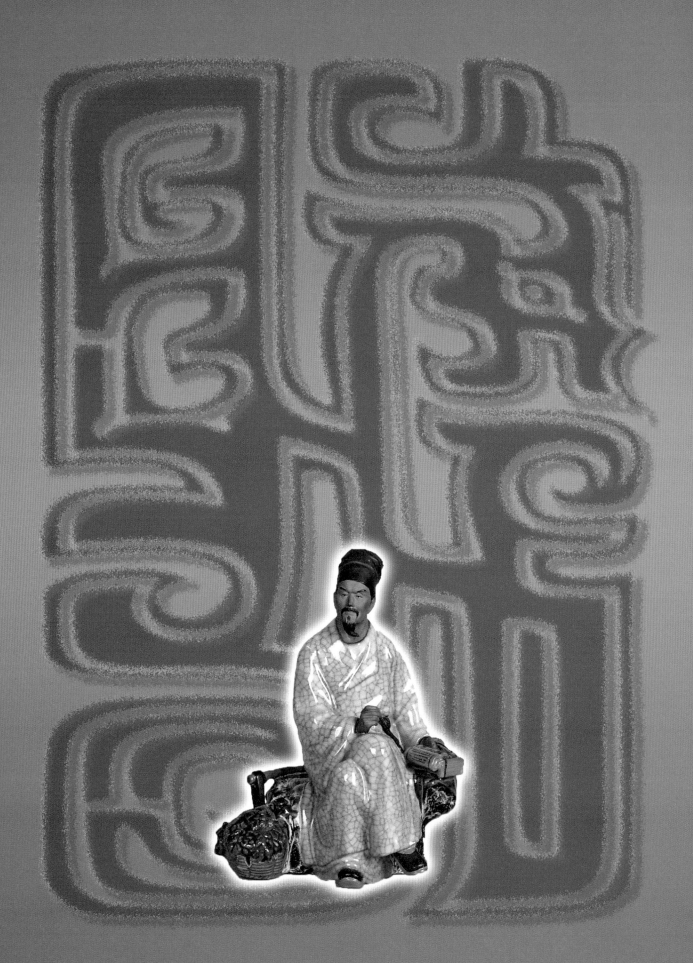

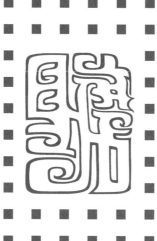

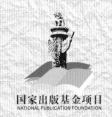

国家出版基金项目
NATIONAL PUBLICATION FOUNDATION

中华医药卫生

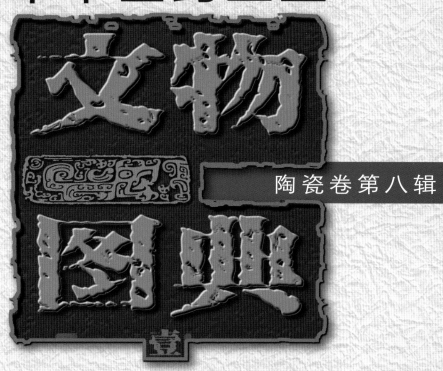

陶瓷卷第八辑

主　编　李经纬　梁　峻　刘学春
总主译　白永权
主　译　杜彦龙

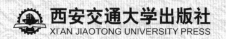

西安交通大学出版社
XI'AN JIAOTONG UNIVERSITY PRESS

图书在版编目 (CIP) 数据

中华医药卫生文物图典 . 1. 陶瓷卷 . 第 8 辑 . / 李经纬，
梁峻，刘学春主编 . — 西安：西安交通大学出版社，2016.12

ISBN 978-7-5605-7035-8

Ⅰ . ①中… Ⅱ . ①李… ②梁… ③刘… Ⅲ . ①中国医药学—
古代陶瓷—中国—图录 Ⅳ . ① R-092 ② K870.2

中国版本图书馆 CIP 数据核字（2015）第 013595 号

书　　名　中华医药卫生文物图典（一）陶瓷卷第八辑

主　　编　李经纬　梁　峻　刘学春

责任编辑　郅梦杰

出版发行　西安交通大学出版社

　　　　　（西安市兴庆南路 10 号　邮政编码 710049）

网　　址　http://www.xjtupress.com

电　　话　（029）82668805　82668502（医学分社）

　　　　　（029）82668315（总编办）

传　　真　（029）82668280

印　　刷　中煤地西安地图制印有限公司

开　　本　889mm×1194mm　1/16　　印张　21.5　字数　315 千字

版次印次　2017 年 12 月第 1 版　2017 年 12 月第 1 次印刷

书　　号　ISBN 978-7-5605-7035-8

定　　价　680.00 元

读者购书、书店添货、如发现印装质量问题，请通过以下方式联系、调换。

订购热线：（029）82665248　（029）82665249

投稿热线：（029）82668805　（029）82668502

读者信箱：medpress@126.com

铭记感受历史
自信自重自强
书贺
中华医药卫生文物图典问世
陈可冀 谨题
二〇一七年肖

陈可冀　中国科学院院士、国医大师

精修醫藥衛生文物

圖典功著當代

深究岐黃學術思想

淵源惠澤千秋

中華醫藥衛生文物圖典出版誌慶

丁酉孟秋 孫光榮 敬題於北京

孫光荣　国医大师

中華醫藥衛生文物圖典出版

彰顯中醫藥
文化精神

體現中醫藥
歷史價值

歲次丁酉夏　王琦

王琦　国医大师

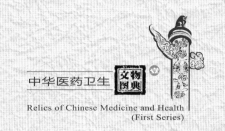

中华医药卫生文物图典（一）
丛书编撰委员会

主　编　李经纬　梁　峻　刘学春

副主编　廖　果　吴鸿洲　康兴军　和中浚　刘小斌　杨金生

　　　　郑怀林　徐江雁　白建疆　黄　煌

编　委　李洪晓　梁永宣　王强虎　董树平　马　健　王　霞

　　　　张雅宗　朱德明　包哈申　张建青　郑　蓉　庄乾竹

　　　　李宏红　刘哲峰　王宏才　陈润东

总主译　白永权

主　译　陈向京　聂文信　范晓晖　温　睿　赵永生　杜彦龙

　　　　吉　乐　李小棉　郭　梦　陈　曦

副主译（按姓氏音序排列）

　　　　董艳云　姜雨孜　李建西　刘　慧　马　健　任宝磊

　　　　任　萌　任　莹　王　颇　习通源　谢皖吉　徐素云

　　　　许崇钰　许　梅　詹菊红　赵　菲　邹郝晶

译　者（按姓氏音序排列）

迟征宇　邓　甜　付一豪　高　琛　高　媛　郭　宁

韩　蕾　何宗昌　胡勇强　黄　鋆　蒋新蕾　康晓薇

李静波　刘雅恬　刘妍萌　鲁显生　马　月　牛笑语

唐云鹏　唐臻娜　田　多　铁红玲　佟健一　王　晨

王　丹　王　栋　王　丽　王　媛　王慧敏　王梦杰

王仙先　吴耀均　席　慧　肖国强　许子洋　闫红贤

杨姣姣　姚　晔　张　阳　张　鋆　张继飞　张梦原

张晓谦　赵　欣　赵亚力　郑　青　郑艳华　朱江嵩

朱瑛培

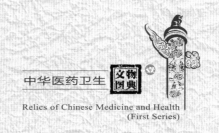

中华医药卫生文物图典

Relics of Chinese Medicine and Health
(First Series)

本册编撰委员会

主　编　李经纬　梁　峻　刘学春

副主编　廖　果　吴鸿洲　康兴军　和中浚　刘小斌　杨金生

　　　　　郑怀林　徐江雁　白建疆　黄　煌

编　委　李洪晓　梁永宣　王强虎　董树平　马　健　王　霞

　　　　　张雅宗　朱德明　包哈申　张建青　郑　蓉　庄乾竹

　　　　　李宏红　刘哲峰　王宏才　陈润东

总主译　白永权

主　译　杜彦龙

副主译　谢皖吉

译　者　康晓薇　刘　慧

丛书策划委员会

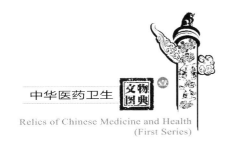

中华医药卫生 文物图典

Relics of Chinese Medicine and Health
(First Series)

序 言

　　探索天、地、人运动变化规律以及"气化物生"过程的相互关系，是人类永恒的课题。宇宙不可逆，地球不可逆，人生不可逆业已成为共识。天地造化形成自然，人类活动构成文化。文物既是文化的载体，又是物化的历史，还是文明的见证。

　　追求健康长寿是人类共同的夙愿。中华民族之所以繁衍昌盛，健康文化起了巨大的推动作用。由于古人谋求生存发展、应对环境变化产生的智慧，大多反映在以医药卫生为核心的健康文化之中，所以，习总书记说："中医药学是中国古代科学的瑰宝，也是打开中华文明宝库的钥匙"。

　　秉持文化大发展、大繁荣理念，中国中医科学院李经纬、梁峻等为负责人的科研团队在完成科技部"国家重点医药卫生文物收集调研和保护"课题获 2005 年度中华中医药学会科技二等奖基础上，又资鉴"夏商周断代工程""中华文明探源工程"等相关考古成果，用有重要价值的新出土文物置换原拍摄质量较差的文物，适当补充民族医药文物，共精选收载 5000 余件。经西安交通大学出版社申报，《中华医药卫生文物图典（一）》（以下简称《图典》）于 2013 年获得了国家出版基金的资助，并经专业翻译团队翻译，使《图典》得以面世。

　　文物承载的信息多元丰富，发掘解读其中蕴藏的智慧并非易事。医药卫生文物更具有特殊性，除文物的一般属性外，还承载着传统医学发展史迹与促进健康的信息。运用历史唯物主义观察发掘文物信息，善于从生活文物中领悟卫生信息，才能准确解读其功能，也才能诠释其在民生健康中的历史作用，收到以古鉴今之效果。"历史是现实的根源"，任何一个民族都不能割断历史，史料都包含在文化中。"文化是民族的血脉，是人民的精神家园"，文化繁荣才能实现中华民族的伟大复兴。值本《图典》付梓之际，用"梳理文化之脉，必获健康之果"作为序言并和作者、读者共勉！

中央文史研究馆馆员
中国工程院院士　　王永炎
丁酉年仲夏

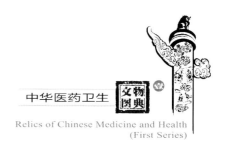

中华医药卫生**文物图典**

Relics of Chinese Medicine and Health
(First Series)

前 言

文化是相对自然的概念，是考古界常用词汇。文物是文化的重要组成部分，既是文明的物证，又是物化的历史。狭义医药卫生文物是疾病防治模式语境下的解读，而广义医药卫生文物则是躯体、心态、环境适应三维健康模式下的诠释。中华民族是 56 个民族组成的多元一体大家庭，中华医药卫生文物当然包括各民族的健康文化遗存。

天地造化如造山、板块漂移、气候变迁、生物起源进化等形成自然。气化物生莫贵于人，即整个生物进化的最高成果是人类自身。广义而言，人类生存思维留下的痕迹即物质财富和精神财富总和构成文化，其一般的物化形式是视觉感知的文物、文献、胜迹等。其中质变标志明晰的文化如文字、文物、城市、礼仪等可称作文明。从唯物史观视角观察，狭义文化即精神财富，尤其体现人类精、气、神状态的事项，其本质也具有特殊物质属性，如量子也具有波粒二相性，这种粒子也是物质，无非运动方式特殊而已。现代所谓可重复验证的"科学"，事实上也是从文化中分离出来的事项，因此也是一种特殊文化形式。追求健康长寿是人类共同的夙愿。中华民族之所以繁衍昌盛，是因为健康文化异彩纷呈。中华优秀传统医药文化之所以博大精深，是因为其原创思维博大、格物致知精深，所以，习总书记说："中医药学是中国古代科学的瑰宝，也是打开中华文明宝库的钥匙"。

文化既反映时代、地域、民族分布、生产资料来源、技术水平等信息，又反映人类认知水平和生存智慧。发掘解读文物、文献中蕴藏的健康知识和灵动智慧，首先是从事健康工作者的责任和义务。《易经》设有"观"卦，人类作为观察者，不仅要积极收藏展陈文物，而且要善于捕捉文物倾诉的信息，汲取养分，启迪思维，收到古为今用之效果。墨子三表法，首先一表即"本之于古者圣王之事"，也是强调古代史实的重要性。"历史是现实的根源"，现实是未来的基础。任何一个国家、地区、民族都不能割断历史、忽略基础，这个基础就是文化。"文化是民族的血脉，是人民的精神家园"。文化繁荣才能驱动各项事业发展，才能实现中华民族的伟大复兴。

人类从类人猿分化出来。"禄丰古猿禄丰种"是云南禄丰发现的类人猿化石，距今七八百万年。距今 200 万年前人类进入旧石器时代，直立行走，打制石器产生工具意识，管理火种，是所谓"燧人氏"时代。中国留存有更新世早、中期的元谋、蓝田、北京人等遗址。距今 10 万—5 万年前，人类进入旧石器时代中期，即早期智人阶段，脑容量增加，和欧洲、非洲人种相比，原始蒙古人种颧骨前突等，是所谓"伏羲氏"时代。中国发现的马坝、长阳、丁村人等较典型。距今 5 万—1 万年前，人类进入旧石器时代晚期，即晚期智人阶段，细石器、骨角器等遍布全国，山顶洞、柳江、资阳人等较典型。

中石器时代距今约 1 万年，是旧石器时代向新石器时代的短暂过渡期，弓箭发明，狗被驯化。河南灵井、陕西沙苑遗址等作为代表。距今 1 万—公元前 2600 年前后，人类进入新石器时代，磨光石器、烧制陶器，出现农业村落并饲养家畜，是所谓"神农氏"时代。公元前 7000 年以来，在甲、骨、陶、石等载体上出现契刻符号、七音阶骨笛乐器等，反映出人文气息趋浓。公元前 6000—公元前 3500 年的老官台、裴李岗、河姆渡、马家浜、仰韶等文化遗址，彰显出先民围绕生存健康问题所做的各种努力。

公元前 4800 年以来，以关中、晋南、豫西为中心形成的仰韶文化，是中原史前文化的重要标志。以半坡、庙底沟类型为典型，自公元前 3500 年走向繁荣，属于锄耕粟黍稻兼营渔猎饲养猪鸡经济方式，彩陶尤其发达。公元前 4400—公元前 3300 年，长江中游的大溪文化，薄胎彩陶和白陶发达。公元前 4300—公元前 2500 年山东丰岛的大汶口文化，红陶为主。公元前 3500 年前后，辽东的红山文化原始宗教发展。公元前 3300 年以来，长江下游由河姆渡、马家浜文化衍续的良渚文化和陇西的马家窑文化、江淮间的薛家岗文化时趋发达。

公元前 2600—公元前 2000 年，黄河中下游龙山文化群形成，冶铸铜器，制作玉器，土坯、石灰、夯筑技术开始应用。公元前 2697 年，轩辕战败炎帝（有说其后裔）、蚩尤而为黄帝纪元元年。黄帝西巡访贤，"至岐见岐伯，引载而归，访于治道"。其引归地"溱洧襟带于前，梅泰环拱于后"，即今河南新密市古城寨。岐黄答问，构建《黄帝内经》健康知识体系，中华文明从关注民生健康起步。颛顼改革宗教，神职人员出现；帝喾修身节用，帝尧和合百国，舜同律度量衡，大禹疏导治水，中华民族不断繁衍昌盛。

公元前 2070 年，禹之子启以豫西晋南为中心建立夏王朝，二里头青铜文化为其特征，半地穴、窑洞、地面建筑并存。饮食卫生器具、酒器增多。朱砂安神作用在宫殿应用。公元前 1600 年，商灭夏。偃师商城设有铸铜作坊。公元前 1300 年，盘庚迁殷，使用甲骨文。武丁时期青铜浑铸、分铸并存。公元前 1056 年，相传周"文王被殷纣拘于羑里，演《周易》，成六十四卦"。公元前 1046 年，武王克商建周，定都镐京。青铜器始铸长篇铭文，周原发掘出微型甲骨文字。公元前 770 年，平王东迁。虢国铸铜柄铁剑。公元前 753 年，秦国设置史官。公元前 707 年出现蝗灾、公元前 613 年出现"哈雷彗星"，均被孔子载入《春秋》。公元前 221 年，秦始皇统一中国，多元一体民族大家庭形成，中华医药卫生文物异彩纷呈。

中国是治史大国，历来重视发展文化博物事业，1955 年成立卫生部中医研究院时就设置医史研究室，1982 年中国医史文献研究所成立时复建中国医史博物馆研究收藏展陈文物。2000—2003 年，经王永炎院士、姚乃礼院长等呼吁，科技部批准立项，由李经纬、梁峻为负责人的团队完成"国家重点医药卫生文物收集调研和保护"项目任务，受到科技部项目验收组专家的高度评价，获中华中医药学会科技进步二等奖。2013 年，在国家出版基金资助下，课题组对部分文物重新拍摄或必要置换、充实民族医药文物后，由西安交通大学出版社编辑、组聘国内一流翻译团队英译说明文字付梓，受到国家中医药博物馆筹备工作领导小组和办公室的高度重视。

"物以类聚"，《图典》主要依据文物质地、种类分为 9 卷，计有陶瓷，金属，纸质，竹木，玉石、织品及标本，壁画石刻及遗址，少数民族文物，其他，备考等卷。同卷下主要根据历史年代或小类分册设章。每卷下的历史时段不求统一。遵循上述规则将《图典》划分为21册，总计收载文物5000余件。对每件文物的描述，除质地、规格、馆藏等基本要素外，重点描述其在民生健康中的作用。对少数暂不明确的事项在括号中注明待考。对引自各博物馆的材料除在文物后列出馆藏外，还在书后再次统一列出馆名或参考书目，以充分尊重其馆藏权，也同时维护本典作者的引用权。

21世纪，围绕人类健康的生命科学将飞速发展，但科学离不开文化，文化离不开文物。发掘文物承载的信息为现实服务，谨引用横渠先生四言之两语："为天地立心，为生民立命"，既作为编撰本《图典》之宗旨，也是我们践行国家"一带一路"倡议的具体努力。希冀通过本《图典》的出版发行，教育国人，提振中华民族精神；走向世界，为人类健康事业贡献力量。

李经纬　梁峻　刘学春

2017年6月于北京

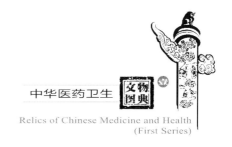

中华医药卫生 文物图典

Relics of Chinese Medicine and Health
(First Series)

目 录

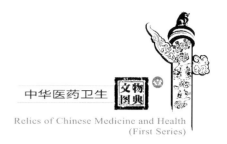

中华医药卫生 文物图典

Relics of Chinese Medicine and Health
(First Series)

Contents

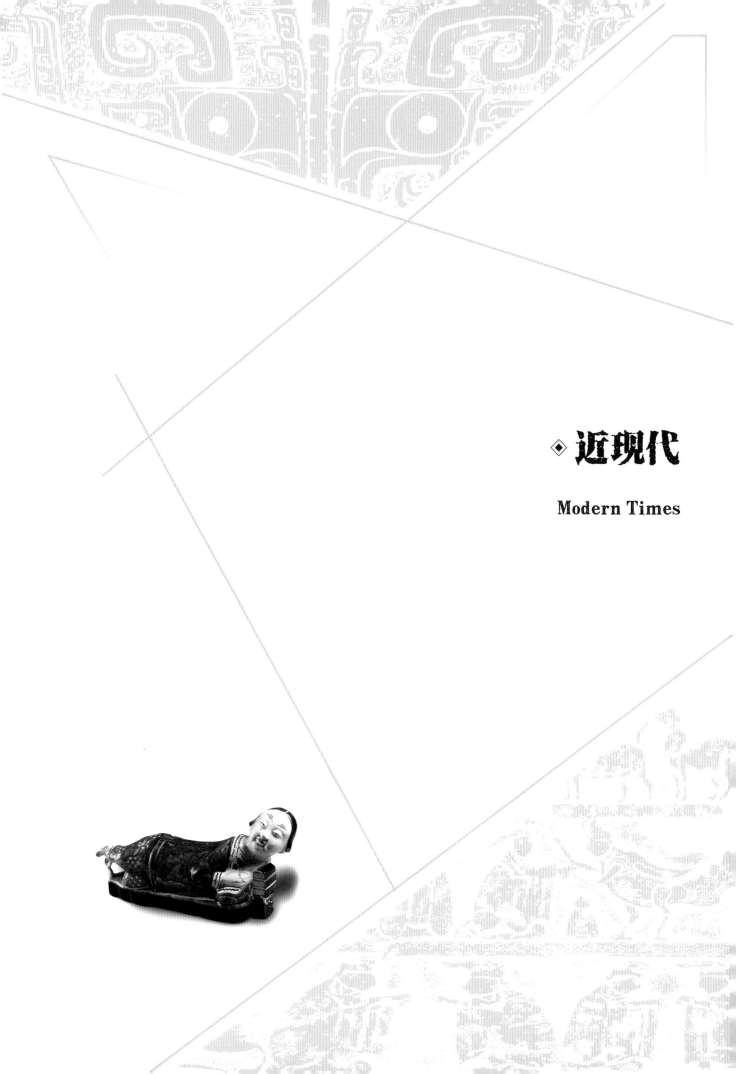

◈ **近现代**

Modern Times

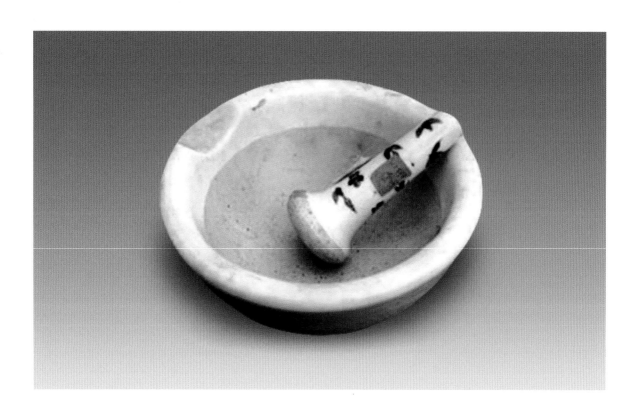

白瓷插钵

现代

瓷质

钵：口外径 15 厘米，底径 8.4 厘米，通高 6.8 厘米，腹深 5.1 厘米，重 1025 克

杵：长 9.5 厘米，重 95 克

Opal Porcelain Mortar and Pestle

Modern Times

Porcelain

Mortar: Mouth Outer Diameter 15 cm/ Bottom Diameter 8.4 cm/ Height 6.8 cm/ Depth 5.1 cm/ Weight 1025 g

Pestle: Length 9.5 cm/ Weight 95 g

带青花杵，钵形似碗，钵口边圆润，钵口有一处外突，形似壶的短流。研细药物用。

广东中医药博物馆藏

The pestle is of blue-and-white porcelain. The mortar is in the shape of a bowl with a round and smooth rim, a small part of which extends outwards like the short spout of a pot. They were utilized for porphyrizing drug ingredients.

Preserved in Guangdong Chinese Medicine Museum

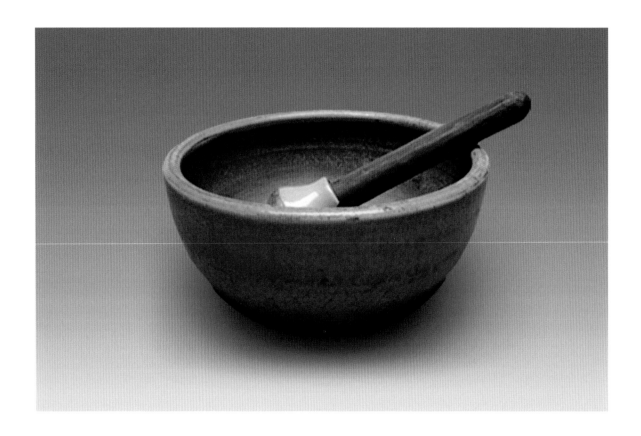

乳钵

民国时期

瓷质

口径 22 厘米，高 10 厘米

Mortar

Republican Period

Porcelain

Mouth Diameter 22 cm/ Height 10 cm

圆口，平底，腹稍内收，器物表面有青色釉，釉上有冰裂纹。由民间征集。

成都中医药大学中医药传统文化博物馆藏

The mortar has a round mouth, a flat bottom and a slightly contracted belly. Its surface is covered with cyan glaze on which are patterns of ice crack. It was collected from a private owner.

Preserved in Museum of Traditional Chinese Medicine Culture, Chengdu University of Traditional Chinese Medicine

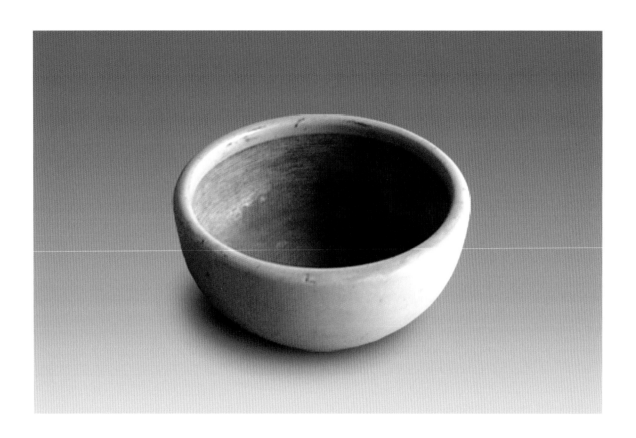

药臼

民国时期

瓷质

口径 14 厘米，高 6 厘米

Medicine Mortar

Republican Period

Porcelain

Mouth Diameter 14 cm/ Height 6 cm

圆口，直腹，平底，外壁施白釉。由民间征集。

成都中医药大学中医药传统文化博物馆藏

The mortar has a round mouth, a straight belly and a flat bottom. The outer wall of the mortar is painted with white glaze. It was collected from a private owner.

Preserved in Museum of Traditional Chinese Medicine Culture, Chengdu University of Traditional Chinese Medicine

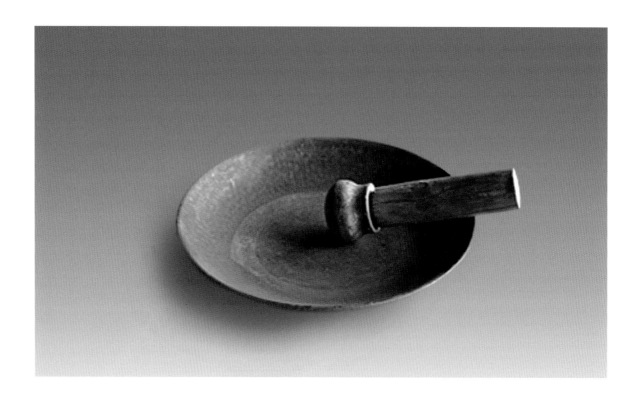

臼

民国时期

瓷质

臼：口径 26 厘米，高 5 厘米

杵：长 16 厘米

Mortar

Republican Period

Porcelain

Mortar: Mouth Diameter 26 cm/ Height 5 cm

Pestle: Length 16 cm

形状类似盘，敞口，圈足，半部施黄釉。由民间征集。

　　成都中医药大学中医药传统文化博物馆藏

The dish-shaped mortar has a flared mouth and a circular foot. Part of its surface is painted with yellow glaze. It was collected from a private owner.

Preserved in Museum of Traditional Chinese Medicine Culture, Chengdu University of Traditional Chinese Medicine

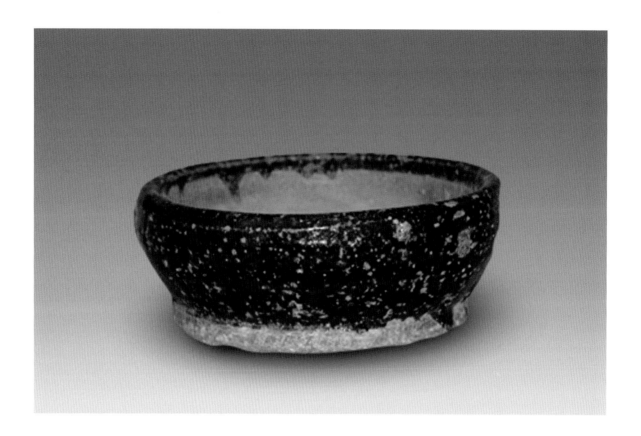

黑釉研钵

近代

瓷质

口径 21 厘米，底径 17 厘米，通高 8 厘米，重 1600 克

Black Glazed Mortar

Modern Times

Porcelain

Mouth Diameter 21 cm/ Bottom Diameter 17 cm/ Height 8 cm/ Weight 1600 g

束口，圆腹，黑釉，比较粗糙。研药工具，有裂印。

陕西医史博物馆藏

Covered with black glaze, the mortar has a contracted mouth and a round belly. Having cracks in it, the mortar is a little bit rough. It was utilized for porphyrizing medical herbs.

Preserved in Shaanxi Museum of Medical History

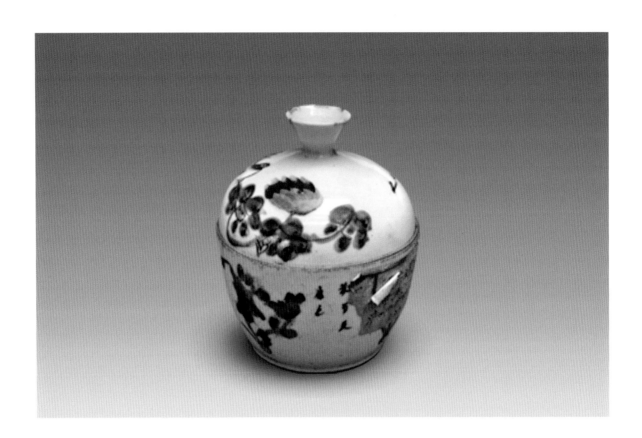

药缸

民国时期

瓷质

口径 10.5 厘米，高 12 厘米

Medicine Jar

Republican Period

Porcelain

Mouth Diameter 10.5 cm/ Height 12 cm

平底，腹内收，杯形盖，上有圈足形纽，盖
与身子母口相合。饰彩色人物图案。由民间
征集。

成都中医药大学中医药传统文化博物馆藏

The jar has a flat bottom and a contracted belly.
The cover, in the shape of a cup and with a ring-
foot handle on top, fits the body of the jar
perfectly well. The jar is decorated with the
design of colorful figures, It was collected
from a private owner.
Preserved in Museum of Traditional Chinese
Medicine Culture, Chengdu University of
Traditional Chinese Medicine

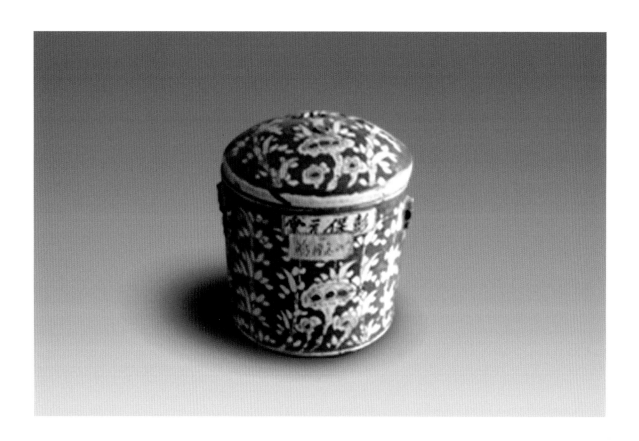

药缸

近代

瓷质

口径 18 厘米，高 20 厘米

Medicine Jar

Modern Times

Porcelain

Mouth Diameter 18 cm/ Height 20 cm

器身或圆桶形，平底，有两个圆形贯耳，盖为穹隆状，上方有把，已残。腹上部有"彭保元堂"铭。由民间征集。

成都中医药大学中医药传统文化博物馆藏

The jar has a cylindrical body, a flat bottom and two circular pierced handles. Its cover is in the shape of vault with a damaged knob on the top. Its belly is inscribed with the Chinese characters "Peng Bao Yuan Tang", meaning the name of the drugstore. It was collected from a private owner.

Preserved in Museum of Traditional Chinese Medicine Culture, Chengdu University of Traditional Chinese Medicine

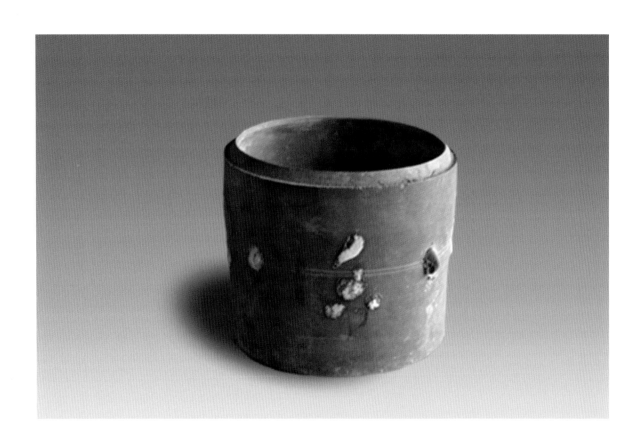

药缸

近代

陶质

口径 11.5 厘米，高 10 厘米

Medicine Jar

Modern Times

Pottery

Mouth Diameter 11.5 cm/ Height 10 cm

圆直筒形。应有盖，惜已残，平底。腹部有
三个贯耳和两道旋纹。由民间征集。

　　成都中医药大学中医药传统文化博物馆藏

The cylindrical jar has three pierced handles,
two strips of spiral patterns on its belly
and a flat bottom. It had a cover which was
unfortunately damaged. It was collected from
a private owner.

Preserved in Museum of Traditional Chinese
Medicine Culture, Chengdu University of
Traditional Chinese Medicine

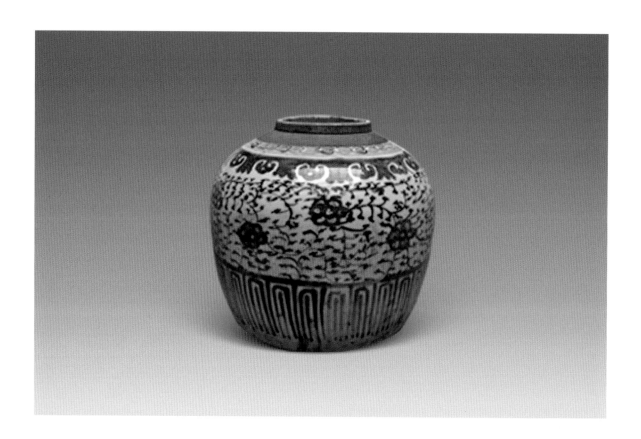

药坛

民国时期

瓷质

底径 17 厘米，高 20 厘米

Medicine Jar

Republican Period

Porcelain

Bottom Diameter 17 cm/ Height 20 cm

平底。腹中上部饰青花缠枝纹，底部饰青花
回文，保存完好。由民间征集。

　　成都中医药大学中医药传统文化博物馆藏

The jar has a flat bottom. The upper part of
its belly is decorated with blue-and-white
flowers in entwining patterns while the
lower part is painted with blue-and-white
meandering designs. The jar still in good
condition. It was collected from a private
owner.

Preserved in Museum of Traditional Chinese
Medicine Culture, Chengdu University of
Traditional Chinese Medicine

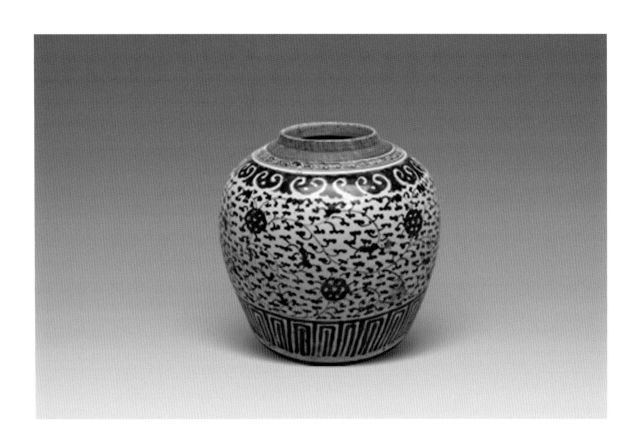

药坛

民国时期

瓷质

底径 17 厘米，高 20 厘米

Medicine Jar

Republican Period

Porcelain

Bottom Diameter 17 cm/ Height 20 cm

平底。腹中上部饰青花缠枝纹，底部饰青花
回文，保存完好。由民间征集。

　　成都中医药大学中医药传统文化博物馆藏

The jar has a flat bottom. The upper part of
its belly is decorated with blue-and-white
flowers in entwining patterns while the
lower part is painted with blue-and-white
meandering designs. The jar still in good
condition. It was collected from a private
owner.

Preserved in Museum of Traditional Chinese
Medicine Culture, Chengdu University of
Traditional Chinese Medicine

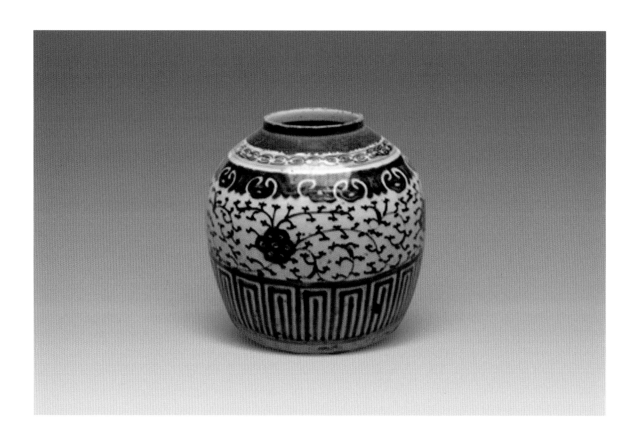

药坛

民国时期

瓷质

口径 9 厘米，底径 12 厘米，高 20 厘米

Medicine Jar

Republican Period

Porcelain

Mouth Diameter 9 cm/ Bottom Diameter 12 cm/ Height 20 cm

鼓腹，平底。腹中上部饰青花缠枝纹，底部
饰青花图纹，保存完好。由民间征集。

成都中医药大学中医药传统文化博物馆藏

The jar has a bulging belly and a flat bottom.
The upper part of its belly is decorated with
blue-and-white flowers in entwining patterns
while the lower part is painted with blue-
and-white meandering designs. The jar still
in good condition. It was collected from a
private owner.

Preserved in Museum of Traditional Chinese
Medicine Culture, Chengdu University of
Traditional Chinese Medicine

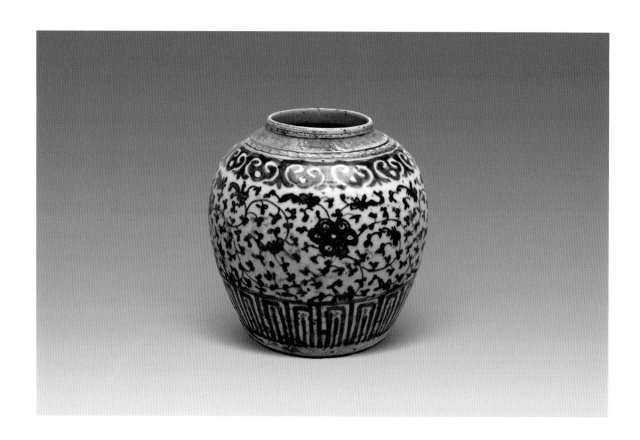

药坛

民国时期

瓷质

口径 9 厘米，底径 17 厘米，高 20 厘米

Medicine Jar

Republican Period

Porcelain

Mouth Diameter 9 cm/ Bottom Diameter 17 cm/ Height 20 cm

直口，鼓腹，平底。腹中上部饰青花缠枝纹，

底部饰青花回纹，保存完好。由民间征集。

成都中医药大学中医药传统文化博物馆藏

The jar has a straight mouth, a bulging belly
and a flat bottom. The upper part of its belly
is decorated with blue-and-white flowers
in entwining patterns while the lower part
is painted with blue-and-white meandering
designs. The jar still in good condition. It was
collected from a private owner.

Preserved in Museum of Traditional Chinese
Medicine Culture, Chengdu University of
Traditional Chinese Medicine

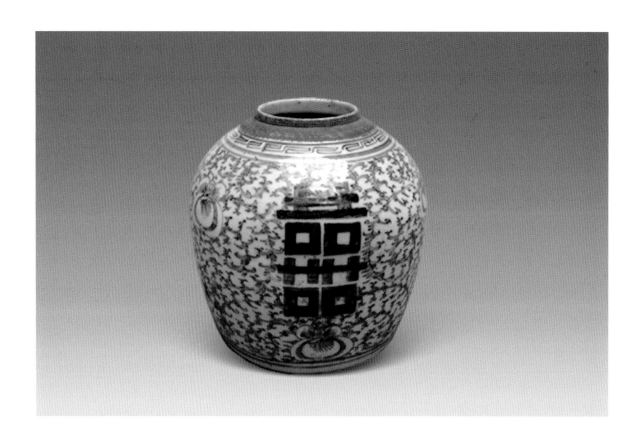

药坛

民国时期

瓷质

口径 19 厘米，底径 17 厘米，高 20 厘米

Medicine Jar

Republican Period

Porcelain

Mouth Diameter 19 cm/ Bottom Diameter 17 cm/ Height 20 cm

直口，鼓腹，平底。遍身饰青花缠枝纹，再在其上饰青花双喜字，保存完好。由民间征集。

成都中医药大学中医药传统文化博物馆藏

The jar has a straight mouth, a bulging belly and a flat bottom, and is decorated with the blue-and-white flowers in entwining patterns on which are written double blue-and-white characters "xi", meaning "double happiness". The jar still in good condition and It was collected from a private owner.

Preserved in Museum of Traditional Chinese Medicine Culture, Chengdu University of Traditional Chinese Medicine

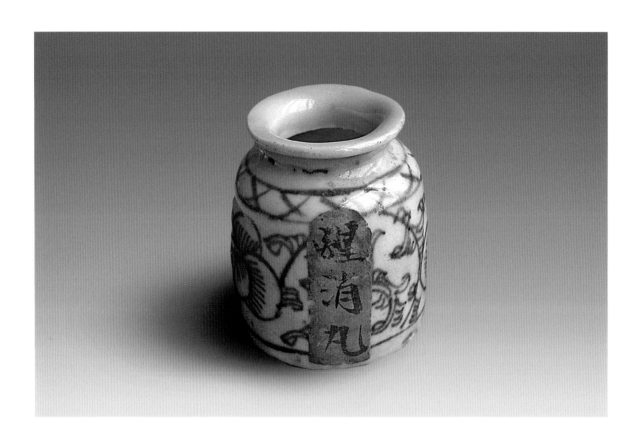

瓷药坛

近代

瓷质

口径 4.1 厘米，腹宽 5 厘米，高 6.2 厘米

Porcelain Medicine Jar

Modern Times

Porcelain

Mouth Diameter 4.1 cm/ Belly Width 5 cm/ Height 6.2 cm

青花小药坛。有"醒消丸"标贴。

江苏省中医药博物馆藏

The small jar is decorated with blue-and-white flowers and labeled with the name of the drug "Xing Xiao Wan".
Preserved in Jiangsu Museum of Traditional Chinese Medicine

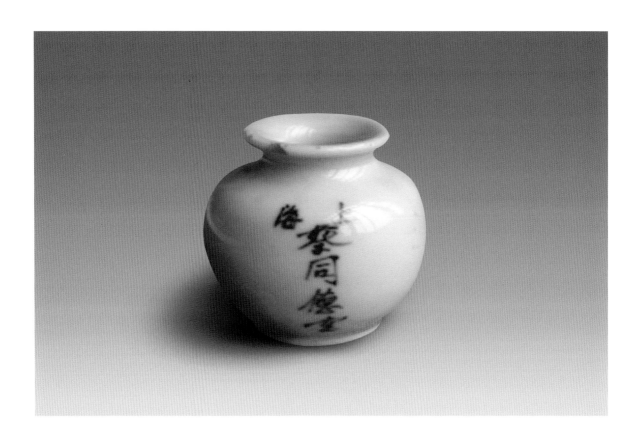

瓷药坛

近代

瓷质

口径 3 厘米，腹宽 4.4 厘米，高 4.9 厘米

Porcelain Medicine Jar

Modern Times

Porcelain

Mouth Diameter 3 cm/ Belly Width 4.4 cm/ Height 4.9 cm

正面有"上海蔡同德堂"等字样，背面有"神效癣药"字样。

江苏省中医药博物馆藏

The jar is inscribed with the name of the drugstore "Shang Hai Cai Tong De Tang" on its obverse side and the brand name of the drug "Shen Xiao Xian Yao" for curing tinea on its reverse side.

Preserved in Jiangsu Museum of Traditional Chinese Medicine

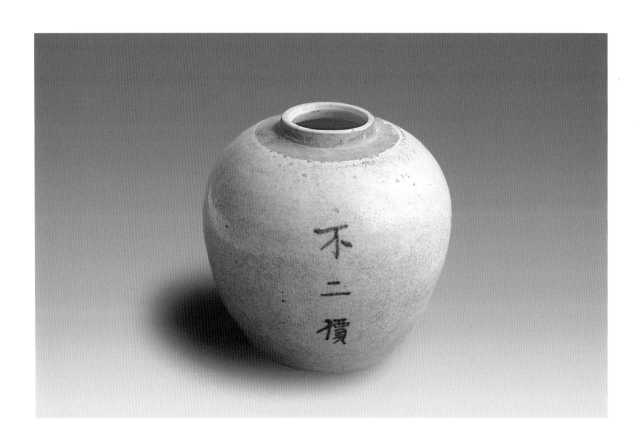

瓷药坛

近代

瓷质

口径 3.5 厘米，腹宽 11.2 厘米，高 11 厘米

有"不二价"等字样。

江苏省中医药博物馆藏

Porcelain Medicine Jar

Modern Times

Porcelain

Mouth Diameter 3.5 cm/ Belly Width 11.2 cm/ Height 11 cm

The jar is inscribed with the Chinese characters "Bu Er Jia" on its surface, meaning fixed price.

Preserved in Jiangsu Museum of Traditional Chinese Medicine

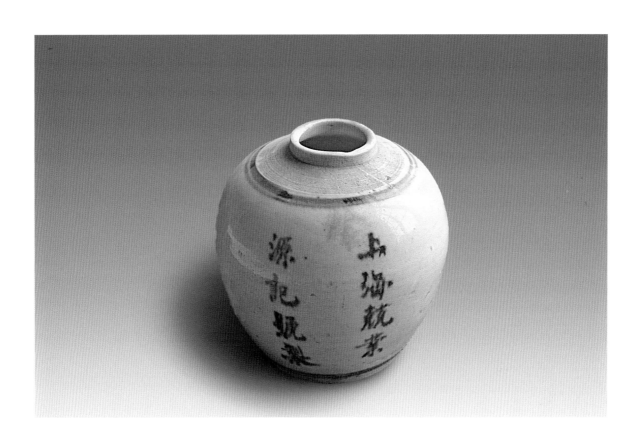

药坛

近代

瓷质

口径3.6厘米，腹宽12厘米，高12.2厘米

有"上海兢业源记号制"字样。

江苏省中医药博物馆藏

Medicine Jar

Modern Times

Porcelain

Mouth Diameter 3.6 cm/ Belly Width 12 cm/

Height 12.2 cm

The jar is inscribed with the Chinese characters

"Shang Hai Jing Ye Yuan Ji Hao Zhi" on its surface,

meaning "Produced by Shanghai Jingyeyuan".

Preserved in Jiangsu Museum of Traditional

Chinese Medicine

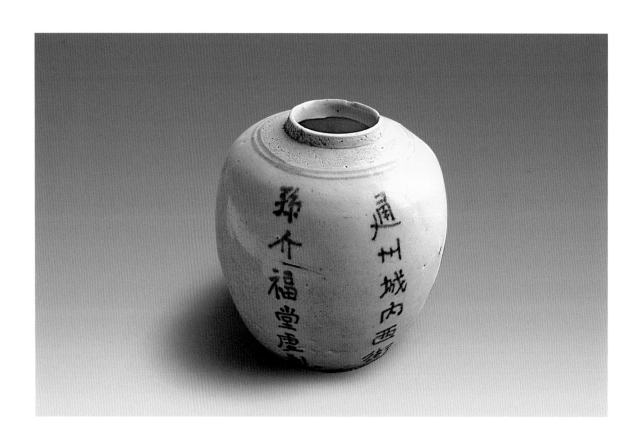

药坛

近代

瓷质

口径 4 厘米，腹宽 11.2 厘米，高 13 厘米

有"通州城内西街孙介福堂处制"字样。

江苏省中医药博物馆藏

Medicine Jar

Modern Times

Porcelain

Mouth Diameter 4 cm/ Belly Width 11.2 cm/ Height 13 cm

The jar is inscribed with the Chinese characters "Tong Zhou Cheng Nei Xi Jie Sun Jie Fu Tang Chu Zhi", meaning the address of the pharmaceutical factory.

Preserved in Jiangsu Museum of Traditional Chinese Medicine

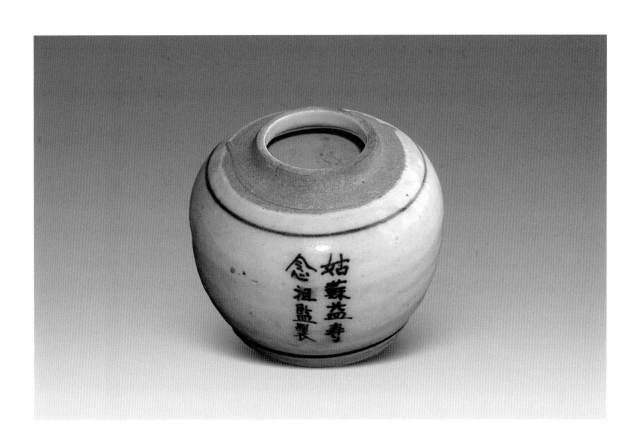

药坛

近代

瓷质

口径 3.8 厘米，腹宽 10 厘米，高 8.6 厘米

有"姑苏益寿念祖监制"字样。

江苏省中医药博物馆藏

Medicine Jar

Modern Times

Porcelain

Mouth Diameter 3.8 cm/ Belly Width 10 cm/ Height 8.6 cm

The jar is inscribed with the Chinese characters "Gu Su Yi Shou Nian Zu Jian Zhi" on its surface, meaning the name of the pharmaceutical factory.

Preserved in Jiangsu Museum of Traditional Chinese Medicine

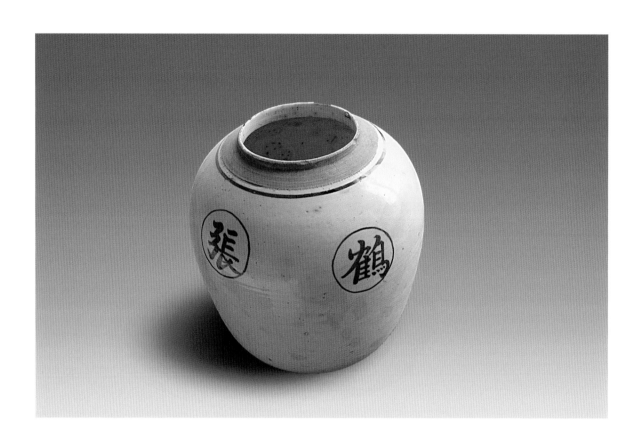

药坛

近代

瓷质

口径 9 厘米，腹宽 20 厘米，高 21 厘米

有"张鹤年"等字样。

江苏省中医药博物馆藏

Medicine Jar

Modern Times

Porcelain

Mouth Diameter 9 cm/ Belly Width 20 cm/ Height 21 cm

The jar is inscribed with the Chinese characters "Zhang He Nian" on its surface, meaning the name of the producer.

Preserved in Jiangsu Museum of Traditional Chinese Medicine

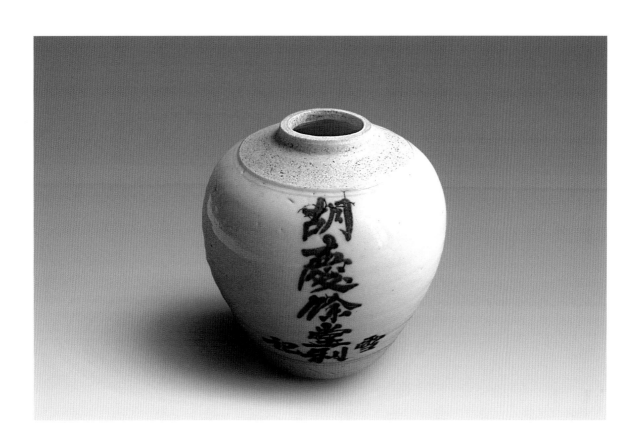

瓷药坛

近代

瓷质

口径 3 厘米，腹宽 9.7 厘米，高 10.3 厘米

有"胡庆馀堂""雪利记"等字样。

江苏省中医药博物馆藏

Porcelain Medicine Jar

Modern Times

Porcelain

Mouth Diameter 3 cm/ Belly Width 9.7 cm/ Height 10.3 cm

The jar is inscribed with the Chinese characters "Hu Qing Yu Tang" and "Xue Li Ji" on its surface, meaning the name of the producer.

Preserved in Jiangsu Museum of Traditional Chinese Medicine

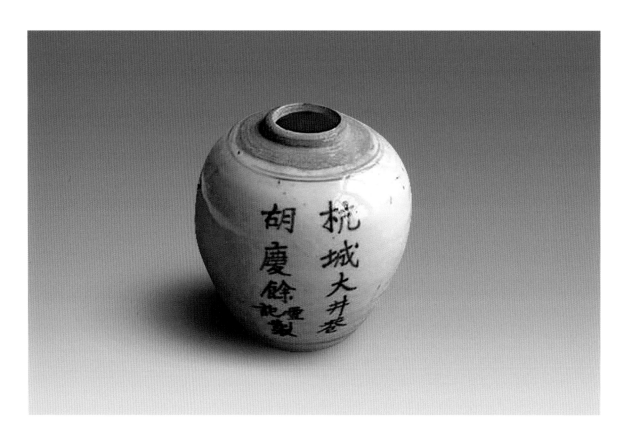

瓷药坛

近代

瓷质

口径 3 厘米，腹宽 9 厘米，高 10.3 厘米

有"杭城大井巷""胡庆馀堂""雪利记"等字样。

江苏省中医药博物馆藏

Porcelain Medicine Jar

Modern Times

Porcelain

Mouth Diameter 3 cm/ Belly Width 9 cm/ Height 10.3 cm

The jar is inscribed with the Chinese characters "Hang Cheng Da Jing Xiang", "Hu Qi Yu Tang" and "Xue Li Ji" on its surface, meaning the address of the pharmaceutical factory and the name of the producer, respectively.

Preserved in Jiangsu Museum of Traditional Chinese Medicine

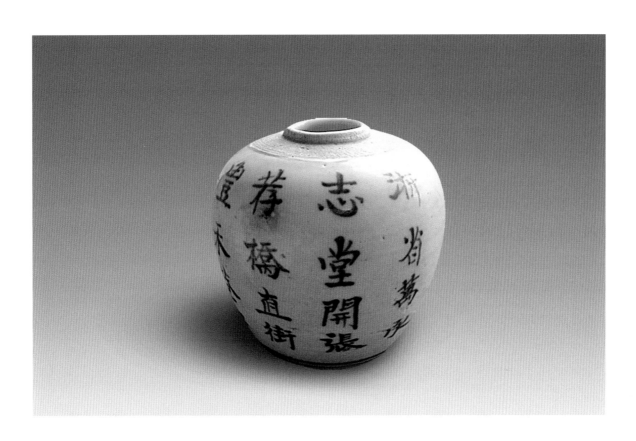

瓷药坛

近代

瓷质

口径 3 厘米，腹宽 9.4 厘米，高 10 厘米

有"浙江省万承志堂开张"等字样。

江苏省中医药博物馆藏

Porcelain Medicine Jar

Modern Times

Porcelain

Mouth Diameter 3 cm/ Belly Width 9.4 cm/ Height 10 cm

The jar is inscribed with the Chinese characters "Zhe Jiang Sheng Wan Cheng Zhi Tang Kai Zhang" on its surface, meaning commemoration of the opening of the drugstore.

Preserved in Jiangsu Museum of Traditional Chinese Medicine

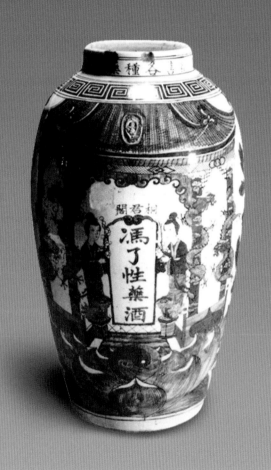

桐君阁药厂药酒坛

清末民初

瓷质

口径 19.7 厘米，高 63 厘米

Medicinal Wine Jar of Tongjunge
Pharmaceutical Factory

Late Qing Dynasty or Early Republican Period
Porcelain
Mouth Diameter 19.7 cm/ Height 63 cm

重庆桐君阁药厂建于 1908 年，是全国有较大影响的中药厂家。此药酒坛直口，半肩腹下渐收，平底，体形硕大。厂名、药酒名称铭记完整。

成都中医药大学中医药传统文化博物馆藏

Tongjunge Pharmaceutical Factory in Chongqing, a greatly influential manufacturer of traditional Chinese medicine, was set up in 1908. The jar has a straight mouth, a flat bottom and a large body which is gradually contracted from its upper belly. The names of the factory and the medicinal wine were inscribed clearly and completely.

Preserved in Museum of Traditional Chinese Medicine Culture, Chengdu University of Traditional Chinese Medicine

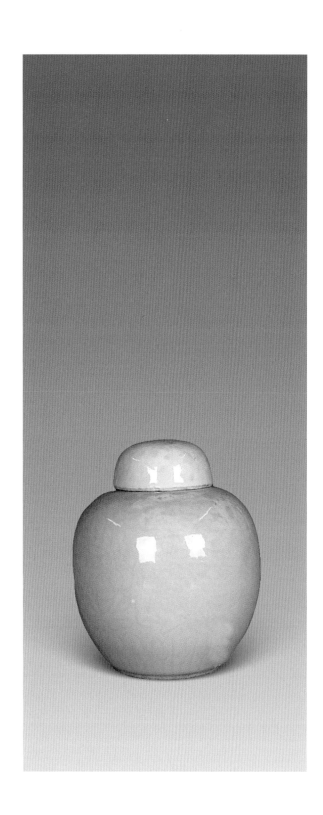

瓷药坛

近现代

瓷质

□内径 4.95 厘米，□外径 5.65 厘米，腹径
13.1 厘米，高 14.6 厘米

Porcelain Medicine Jar

Modern Times

Porcelain

Mouth Inner Diameter 4.95 cm/ Mouth Outer
Diameter 5.65 cm/ Belly Diameter 13.1 cm/
Height 14.6 cm

坛形，施青灰釉，釉下浅刻花草图案，上配扣盖，直口圈足平底，底有"大清雍正年制"款识和"CHINA"浅刻，工艺精细，保存基本完好。盛药用具。1955 年入藏。

中华医学会 / 上海中医药博物馆藏

The jar, for storing medicine, is covered with bluish grey glaze under which patterns of flowers and plants are shallowly carved. It has a cover, a straight mouth, a ring foot and a flat bottom on which is incised an inscription "Da Qing Yong Zheng Nian Zhi" and "CHINA" in shallow carving. The jar is exquisite and is still in good condition. It was collected in the year 1955.

Preserved in Chinese Medical Association/ Museum of Chinese Medicine, Shanghai University of Traditional Chinese Medicine

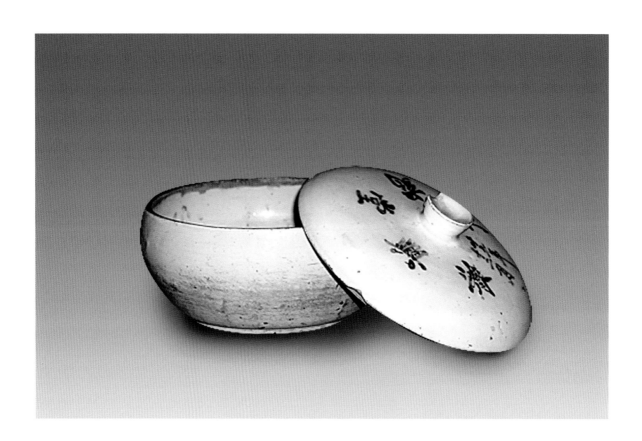

青花药罐

清代民初

瓷质

口径 18 厘米，底径 13 厘米，通高 13 厘米，重 1750 克

Blue-and-white Medicine Pot

Late Qing Dynasty or Early Republican Period

Porcelain

Mouth Diameter 18 cm/ Bottom Diameter 13 cm/ Height 13 cm/ Weight 1750 g

子母口，扁腹，圈足，盖上有"济兴堂药店""三六年十二月"字。盛贮器具，三级文物，完整无损，陕西省济兴堂药店。

陕西医史博物馆藏

The pot has a flat belly, a ring foot and two matching mouths on which the cover is inscribed with the Chinese characters "Ji Xing Tang Yao Dian" and "San Liu Nian Shi Er Yue", meaning the name of the drugstore and the date. It was utilized for storing medicine. It is a third-grade cultural relic and is still in good condition. It was collected from Jixingtang Drugstore in Shaanxi Province.

Preserved in Shaanxi Museum of Medical History

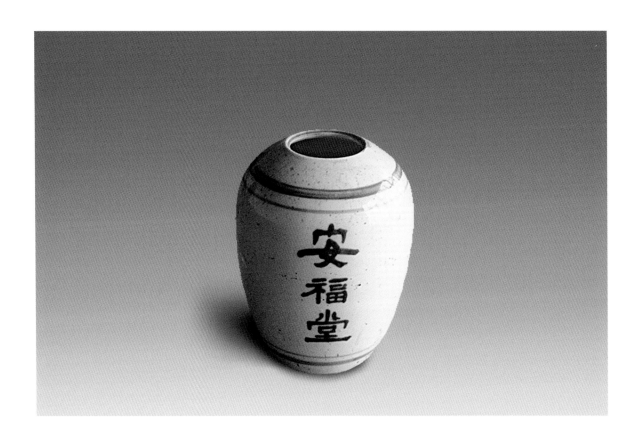

药罐

近代

瓷质

口径 8 厘米，底径 13 厘米，高 24 厘米

Medicine Pot

Modern Times

Porcelain

Mouth Diameter 8 cm/ Bottom Diameter 13 cm/ Height 24 cm

鼓肩，浅圈足，施白釉，腹部有"安福堂"铭。
由民间征集。

　　成都中医药大学中医药传统文化博物馆藏

The pot, painted with white glaze, has a
bulging shoulder and a shallow ring foot. The
belly is inscribed with the Chinese characters
"An Fu Tang", meaning the name of the
drugstore It was collected from a private owner.
Preserved in Museum of Traditional Chinese
Medicine Culture, Chengdu University of
Traditional Chinese Medicine

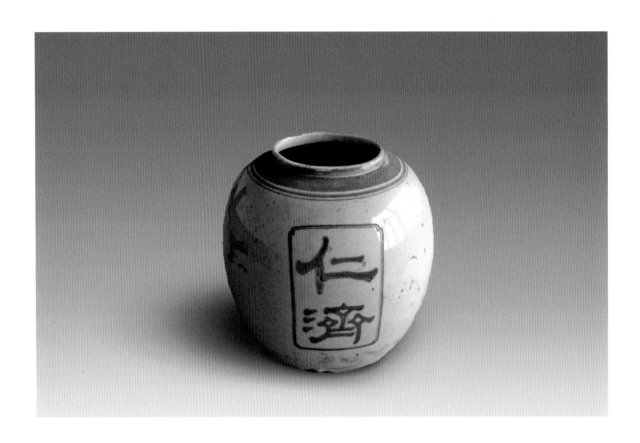

药罐

民国时期

瓷质

口径 12 厘米，高 23 厘米

Medicine Pot

Republican Period

Porcelain

Mouth Diameter 12 cm/ Height 23 cm

器身呈鼓形，平底，施白釉，腹部有"仁济"
二字。由民间征集。

　　成都中医药大学中医药传统文化博物馆藏

The pot, painted with white glaze, has a
bulging body and a flat bottom. Its belly is
inscribed with two Chinese characters "Ren
Ji", meaning the name of the drugstore. It was
collected from a private owner.

Preserved in Museum of Traditional Chinese
Medicine Culture, Chengdu University of
Traditional Chinese Medicine

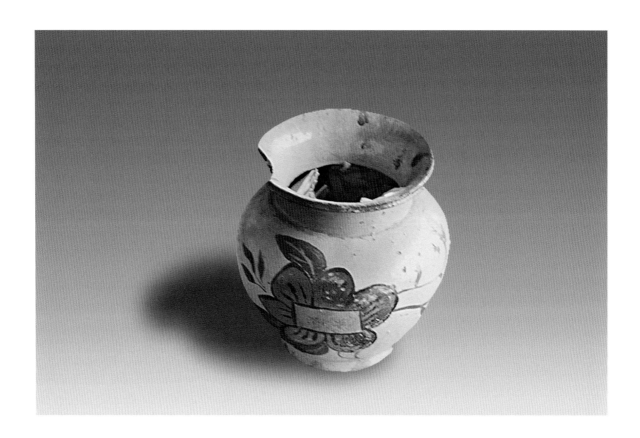

药罐

民国时期

瓷质

口径 11 厘米，高 14 厘米

Medicine Pot

Republican Period

Porcelain

Mouth Diameter 11 cm/ Height 14 cm

口微敞，鼓腹，平底，器身施黄釉。由民间征集。

成都中医药大学中医药传统文化博物馆藏

The pot, painted with yellow glaze, has a flared mouth, a bulging belly and a flat bottom. It was collected from a private owner.

Preserved in Museum of Traditional Chinese Medicine Culture, Chengdu University of Traditional Chinese Medicine

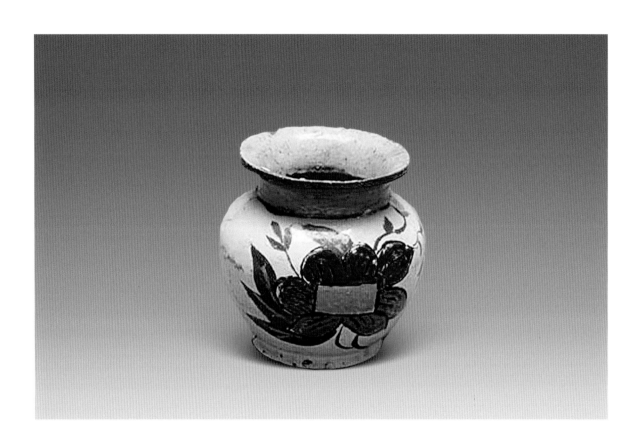

药罐

民国时期

瓷质

口径 11 厘米，高 14 厘米

Medicine Pot

Republican Period

Porcelain

Mouth Diameter 11 cm/ Height 14 cm

口微敞，鼓腹，平底，器身施黄釉，腹部有
五彩花朵纹。藏族地区的盛药用具。由民间
征集。

成都中医药大学中医药传统文化博物馆藏

The pot, painted with yellow glaze, has
a flared mouth, a bulging belly and a flat
bottom. Its belly is painted with five-color
flower designs. It was one of the medicine
storing tools in Tibetan area. It was collected
from a private owner.

Preserved in Museum of Traditional Chinese
Medicine Culture, Chengdu University of
Traditional Chinese Medicine

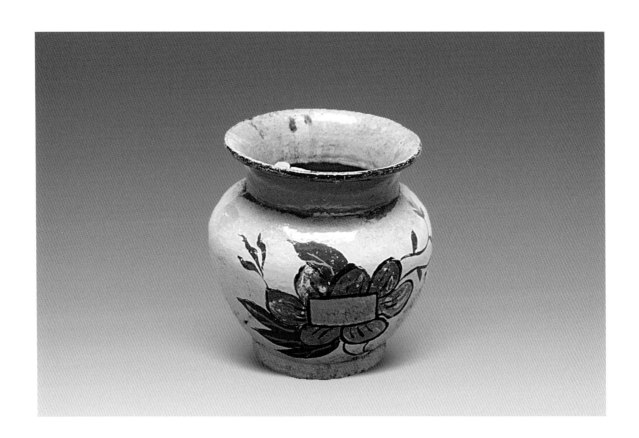

药罐

民国时期

瓷质

口径 11 厘米，高 14 厘米

Medicine Pot

Republican Period

Porcelain

Mouth Diameter 11 cm/ Height 14 cm

口微敞，鼓腹，平底，器身施黄釉，腹部有
五彩花朵纹。藏族地区的盛药用具。由民间
征集。

成都中医药大学中医药传统文化博物馆藏

The pot, painted with yellow glaze, has
a flared mouth, a bulging belly and a flat
bottom. Its belly is painted with five-color
flower designs. It was one of the medicine
storing tools in Tibetan area. It was collected
from a private owner.

Preserved in Museum of Traditional Chinese
Medicine Culture, Chengdu University of
Traditional Chinese Medicine

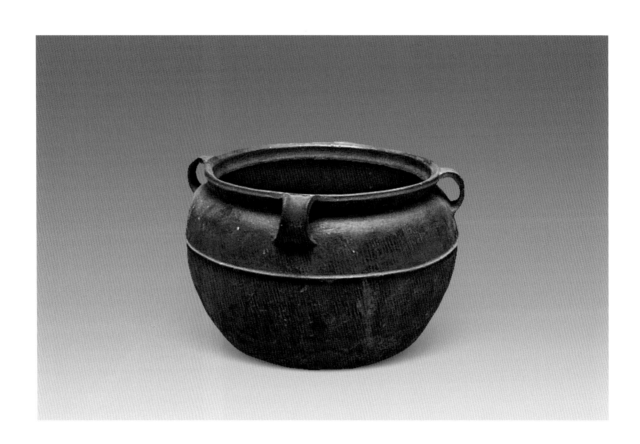

药罐

民国时期

陶质

口径 24 厘米，高 19 厘米

Medicine Pot

Republican Period

Pottery

Mouth Diameter 24 cm/ Height 19 cm

束颈，鼓肩，平底，肩腹部有一道旋纹，四个板桥形耳。熬制药物的工具。由民间征集。

成都中医药大学中医药传统文化博物馆藏

The pot has a contracted neck, a bulging shoulder, a flat bottom and four slab bridge-shaped handles. Its belly is painted with a strip of spiral patterns. It was utilized for decocting Chinese herbs and was collected from a private owner.

Preserved in Museum of Traditional Chinese Medicine Culture, Chengdu University of Traditional Chinese Medicine

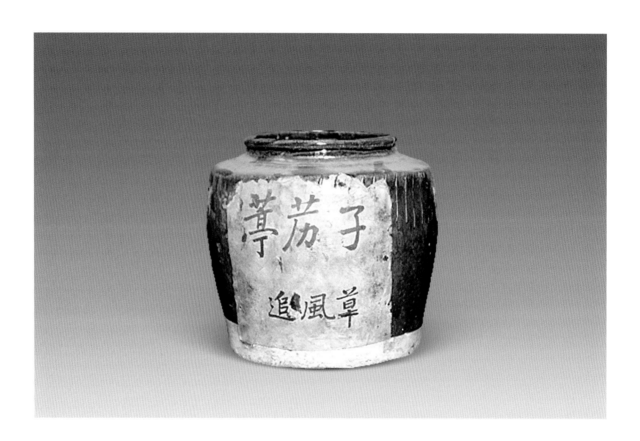

黑瓷罐

近代

瓷质

口径 13 厘米，底径 16.5 厘米，通高 18 厘米，重 1550 克

Black Porcelain Pot

Modern Times

Porcelain

Mouth Diameter 13 cm/ Bottom Diameter 16.5 cm/ Height 18 cm/ Weight 1550 g

圆唇，平肩，直腹，平底，下腹一寸高处白胎无釉。
盛贮器。完整无损。

陕西医史博物馆藏

The pot has a round rim, a flat shoulder, a straight
belly and a flat bottom. One inch from the lower
belly is unglazed and white body. It is still in
good condition.

Preserved in Shaanxi Museum of Medical History

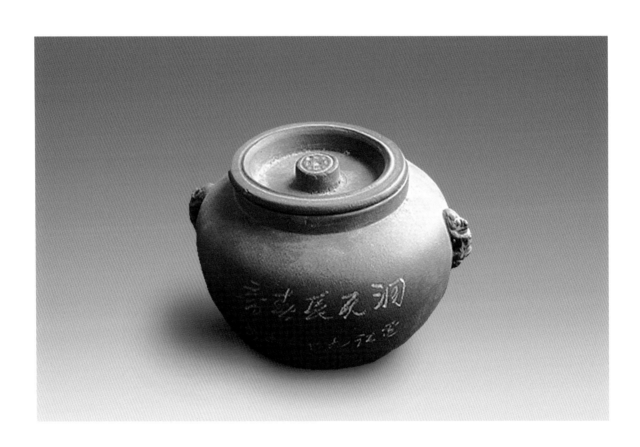

紫砂药罐

近代

紫砂

口径 5.4 厘米，腹宽 10.2 厘米，高 6.7 厘米

有"洞天长春膏""电话九七二九四"等字样。

江苏省中医药博物馆藏

Red Porcelain Medicine Pot

Modern Times

Red Porcelain

Mouth Diameter 5.4 cm/ Belly Width 10.2 cm/ Height 6.7 cm

The pot is inscribed with the Chinese characters "Dong Tian Chang Chun Gao" and "Dian Hua Jiu Qi Er Jiu Si", meaning the name of the drug and the telephone number of the drugstore, respectively.

Preserved in Jiangsu Museum of Traditional Chinese Medicine

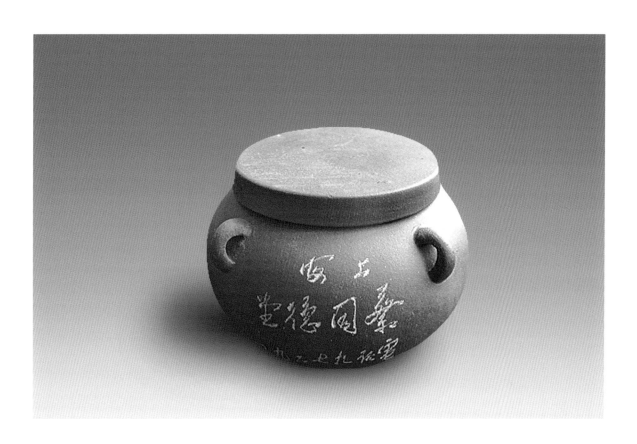

紫砂药罐

近代

紫砂

口径 5.3 厘米，腹宽 10.6 厘米，高 6.7 厘米

四耳紫砂药罐。有"上海蔡同德堂""电话九七二九四"等字样。

江苏省中医药博物馆藏

Red Porcelain Medicine Pot

Modern Times

Red Porcelain

Mouth Diameter 5.3 cm/ Belly Width 10.6 cm/ Height 6.7 cm

The pot has four handles and is inscribed with the Chinese characters "Shang Hai Cai Tong De Tang"and "Dian Hua Jiu Qi Er Jiu Si", meaning the name and the telephone number of the drugstore.

Preserved in Jiangsu Museum of Traditional Chinese Medicine

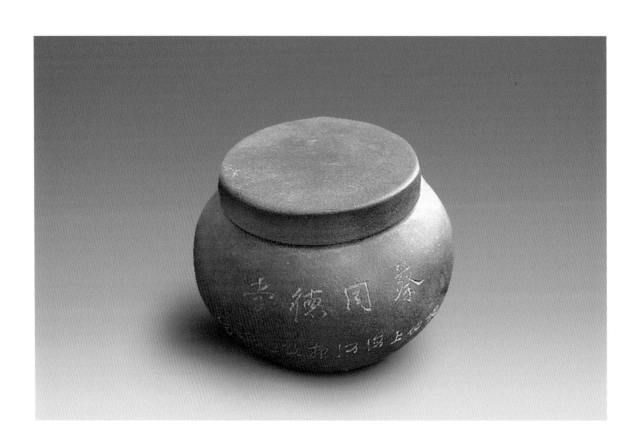

紫砂药罐

近代

紫砂

口径 5.3 厘米，腹宽 10.6 厘米，高 7 厘米

有"蔡同德堂"等字样。

江苏省中医药博物馆藏

Red Porcelain Medicine Pot

Modern Times

Red Porcelain

Mouth Diameter 5.3 cm/ Belly Width 10.6 cm/ Height 7 cm

The pot is inscribed with the Chinese characters "Cai Tong De Tang", meaning the name of the drugstore.

Preserved in Jiangsu Museum of Traditional Chinese Medicine

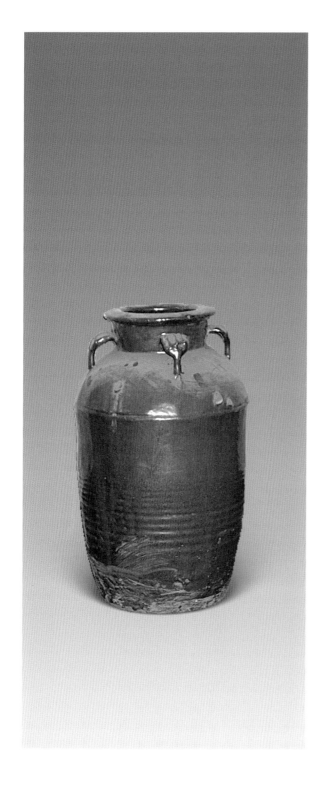

大瓷药罐

近代

瓷质

口径 24 厘米，底径 25 厘米，通高 60 厘米

平敞口，直颈，圆肩，直腹，平底，四耳，淡棕色。盛贮器，完整无损。河南省征集。

陕西医史博物馆藏

Big Porcelain Medicine Gallipot

Modern Times

Porcelain

Mouth Diameter 24 cm/ Bottom Diameter 25 cm/ Height 60 cm

The maple-colored pot has a flat and flared mouth, a straight neck, a straight belly, a round shoulder, a flat bottom and four handles. It was utilized for storing medicine. The pot is still in good condition, It was collected from Henan Province.

Preserved in Shaanxi Museum of Medical History

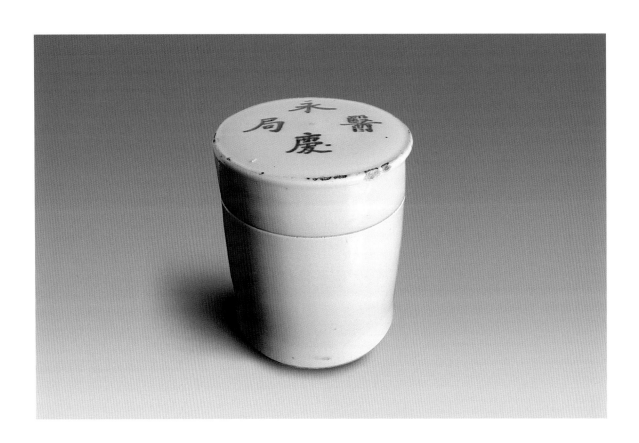

永庆药局药罐

民国时期

瓷质

直径 12 厘米，高 13.5 厘米

Medicine Pot of Yongqing Pharmacy

Republican Period

Porcelain

Diameter 12 cm/ Height 13.5 cm

民国时期，绍兴朱阆仙在绍兴东昌坊设永庆医局，专治跌打损伤。

朱德明藏

During Republican Period, Zhu Langxian, who was from Shaoxing, set up Yongqing Pharmacy in Dongchang Lane of Shaoxing, specializing in treating traumatic injuries.

Preserved by Zhu Deming

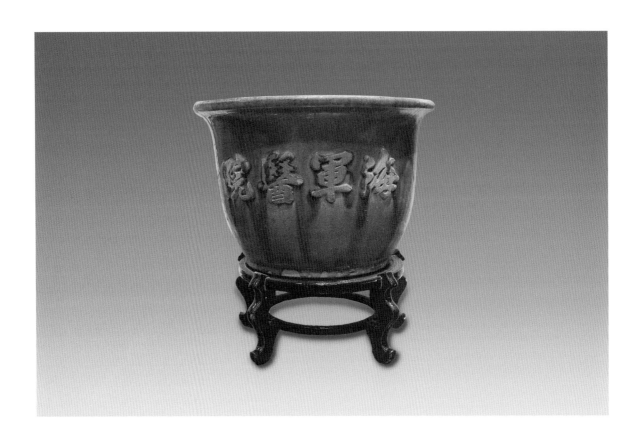

海军医院花盆

民国时期

瓷质

口径 40 厘米，高 30 厘米

Flowerpot of the Naval Hospital

Republican Period

Porcelain

Mouth Diameter 40 cm/ Height 30 cm

圆底，圈足，附木托。整敞口，腹有"海军医院"4
字。民国海军医院（南京）绿釉花盆。

上海医药文献博物馆民国馆藏

The green glazed flowerpot from the Naval
Hospital (Nanjing) in Republican Period has an
open mouth, a round bottom and a ring foot. The
belly is inscribed with four Chinese characters
"Hai Jun Yi Yuan", meaning Naval Hospital.
Preserved in the Museum of the Republic of China,
Shanghai Medical Literature Museum

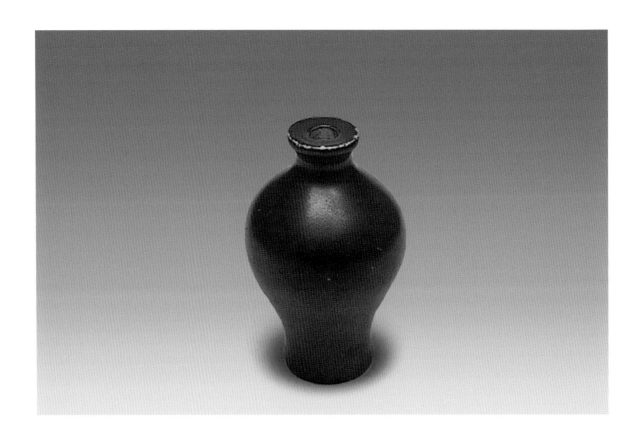

药瓶

民国时期

瓷质

高 6.5 厘米

Medicine Bottle

Republican Period

Porcelain

Height 6.5 cm

束颈，鼓腹，平底。由民间征集。

成都中医药大学中医药传统文化博物馆藏

The bottle has a contracted neck, a bulging belly and a flat bottom. It was collected from a private owner.

Preserved in Museum of Traditional Chinese Medicine Culture, Chengdu University of Traditional Chinese Medicine

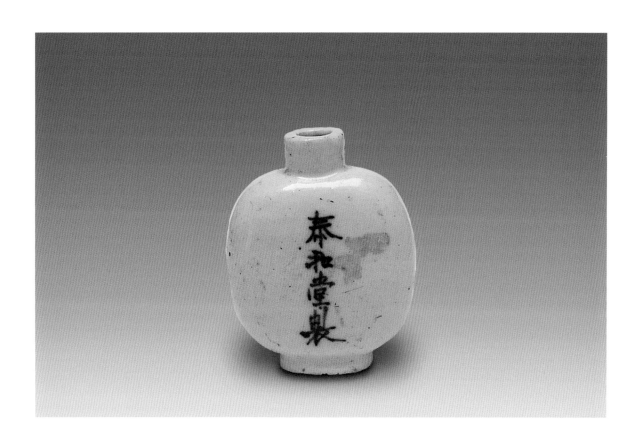

药瓶

民国时期

瓷质

口径 1.8 厘米，底宽 3 厘米，底厚 2 厘米，腹宽 6 厘米，腹厚 2.5 厘米，高 7 厘米

Medicine Bottle

Republican Period

Porcelain

Mouth Diameter 1.8 cm/ Bottom Width 3 cm/ Bottom Thickness 2 cm/ Belly Width 6 cm/ Belly

Thickness 2.5 cm/ Height 7 cm

扁平形，口部呈圆井形，平口直肩，圆鼓形腹，圈足底。腹部书"泰和堂制"文，为盛装小型药物的工具，保存完好。由民间征集。

成都中医药大学中医药传统文化博物馆藏

The cuboid bottle has a round well-shaped mouth, a straight shoulder, a round bulging belly, and a ring foot. Its belly is inscribed with the Chinese characters "Tai He Tang Zhi", meaning produced by Tai He Tang. It was utilized for storing minitype medicine. The bottle is still in good condition. It was collected from a private owner.

Preserved in Museum of Traditional Chinese Medicine Culture, Chengdu University of Traditional Chinese Medicine

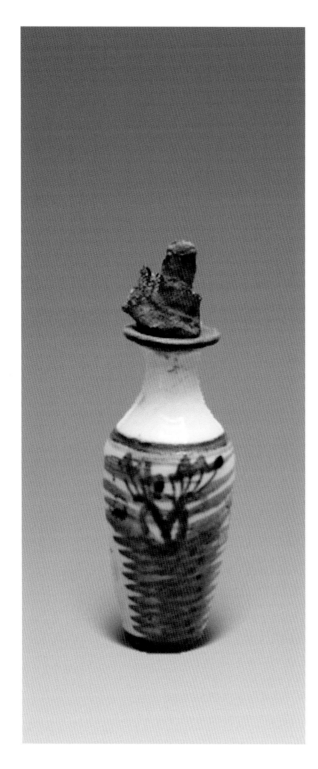

药瓶

民国时期

瓷质

高 14.5 厘米

盘口，细长颈，鼓肩，直腹，平底。饰青花山水纹，保存完好。由民间征集。

　　　成都中医药大学中医药传统文化博物馆藏

Medicine Bottle

Republican Period

Porcelain

Height 14.5 cm

The bottle, decorated with blue-and-white landscape designs, has a dish-shaped mouth, an elongated neck, a bulgy shoulder, a straight belly and a flat bottom. It is still in good condition and was collected from a private owner.

Preserved in Museum of Traditional Chinese Medicine Culture, Chengdu University of Traditional Chinese Medicine

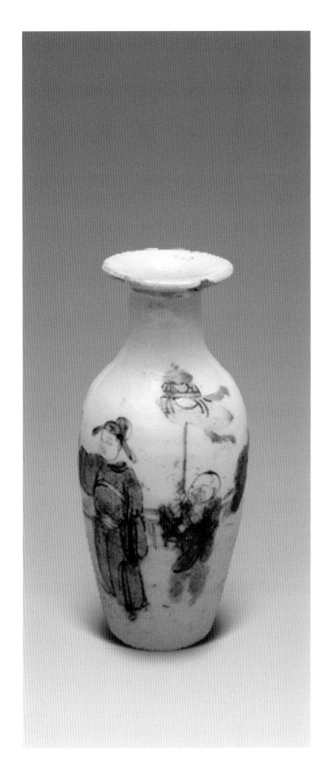

药瓶

民国时期

瓷质

高 14.5 厘米

盘口，细长颈，鼓肩，直腹，平底。饰五彩人物图案，保存完整。由民间征集。

　　　　成都中医药大学中医药传统文化博物馆藏

Medicine Bottle

Republican Period

Porcelain

Height 14.5 cm

The bottle, decorated with the design of five-color figures, has a dish-shaped mouth, an elongated neck, a bulgy shoulder, a straight belly and a flat bottom. It is still in good condition. The bottle collected from a private owner.

Preserved in Museum of Traditional Chinese Medicine Culture, Chengdu University of Traditional Chinese Medicine

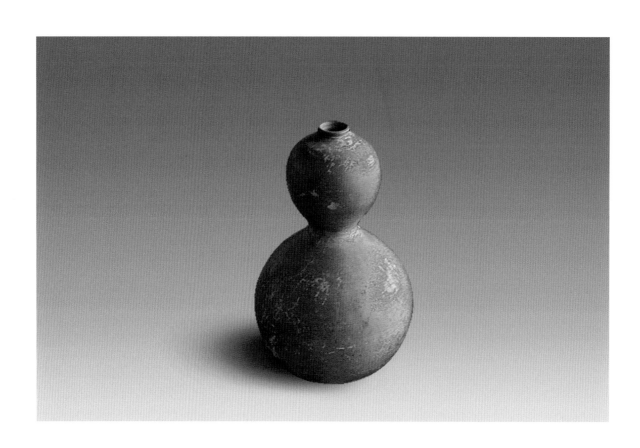

药瓶

近代

陶质

高 16.5 厘米

为葫芦形状，施红釉。由民间征集。

成都中医药大学中医药传统文化博物馆藏

Medicine Bottle

Modern Times

Pottery

Height 16.5 cm

The bottle shaped like a gourd is painted with red glaze. It was collected from a private owner.

Preserved in Museum of Traditional Chinese Medicine Culture, Chengdu University of Traditional Chinese Medicine

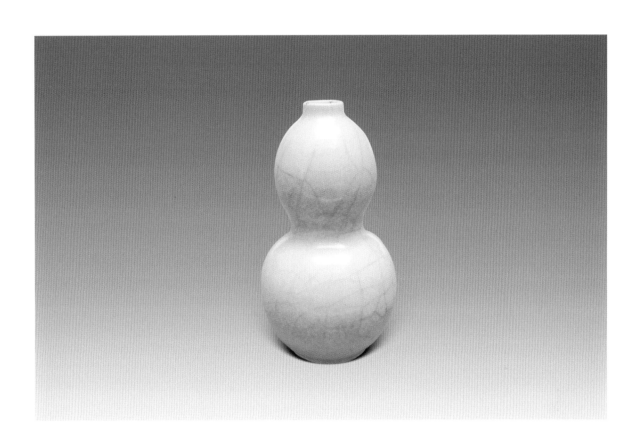

药瓶

民国时期

瓷质

高 25 厘米

状似葫芦，施青釉，有冰裂纹。由民间征集。

　　　成都中医药大学中医药传统文化博物馆藏

Medicine Bottle

Republican Period

Porcelain

Height 25 cm

The bottle shaped like a gourd is painted with green glaze on which are patterns of ice cracks. It was collected from a private owner.

Preserved in Museum of Traditional Chinese Medicine Culture, Chengdu University of Traditional Chinese Medicine

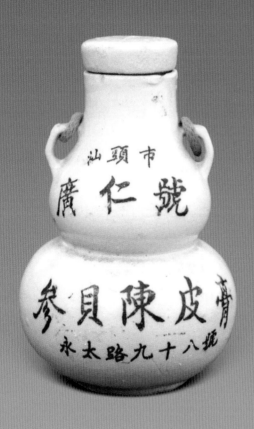

"广仁号" 药瓶

近代

瓷质

高 9.1 厘米

Medicine Bottle with the Brand Guangren

Modern Times

Porcelain

Height 9.1 cm

"广仁号"系近代广东汕头之名中药店，此瓶系该店装贮健脾祛痰之常用中成药参贝陈皮膏的葫芦形药瓶。

广东中医药博物馆藏

Guangren Chinese Medicinal Herbs Shop was one of the famous Chinese medicine herbs shops in Shantou of Guangdong Province in modern times. The gourd-shaped bottle utilized for storing Canbei and Chenpi cream, the common Chinese patent drugs used for tonifying the spleen and eliminating phlegm.

Preserved in Guangdong Chinese Medicine Museum

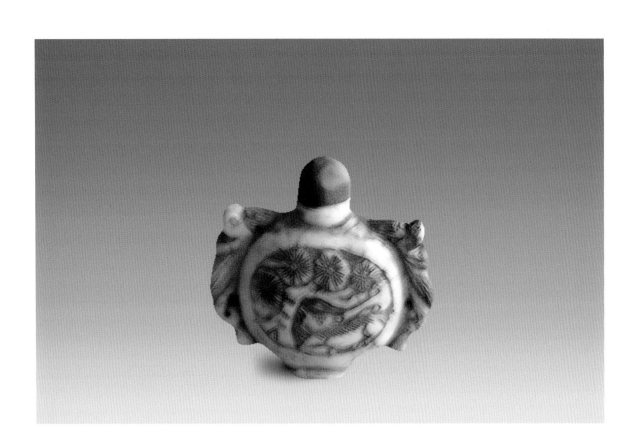

药瓶

民国时期

瓷质

高 6.5 厘米

瓶身较扁，呈鼓形，两侧有堆塑的两翼，圈足。腹部有刻划的花草纹饰。

成都中医药大学中医药传统文化博物馆藏

Medicine Bottle

Republican Period

Porcelain

Height 6.5 cm

The bottle has a flat and bulging body, a ring foot, and two paste-on-paste handles on both sides. Its belly is inscribed with the patterns of flowers and plants.

Preserved in Museum of Traditional Chinese Medicine Culture, Chengdu University of Traditional Chinese Medicine

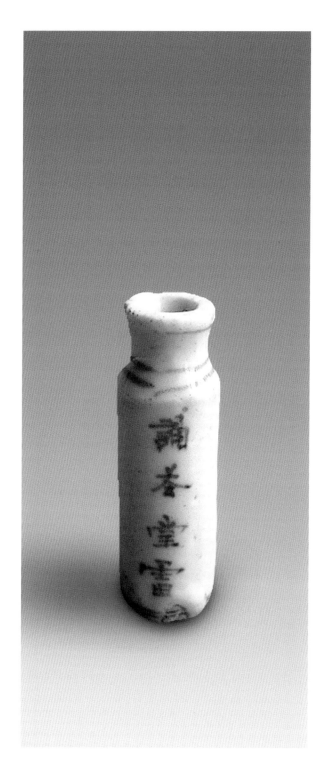

药瓶

近代

瓷质

口径 0.7 厘米，腹宽 1.6 厘米，高 5.3 厘米

立柱形，有"诵苓堂雷"字样。

江苏省中医药博物馆藏

Medicine Bottle

Modern Times

Porcelain

Mouth Diameter 0.7 cm/ Belly Width 1.6 cm/
Height 5.3 cm

The column-shaped bottle is inscribed with
the Chinese characters "Song Ling Tang Lei",
meaning the name of the drugstore.

Preserved in Jiangsu Museum of Traditional
Chinese Medicine

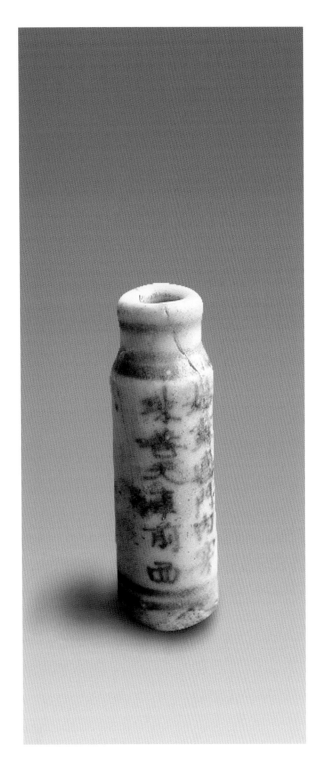

药瓶

近代

瓷质

口径 0.7 厘米，腹宽 1.6 厘米，高 5.3 厘米

立柱形，唇形口，束颈，溜肩，圆圈底，有"姑苏阊门内"等字样。

江苏省中医药博物馆藏

Medicine Bottle

Modern Times

Porcelain

Mouth Diameter 0.7 cm/ Belly Width 1.6 cm/ Height 5.3 cm

The column-shaped bottle has a lip opening, a contracted neck, a smooth shoulder and a round bottom. It is inscribed with the Chinese characters "Gu Su Chang Men Nei", meaning the address of the drugstore.

Preserved in Jiangsu Museum of Traditional Chinese Medicine

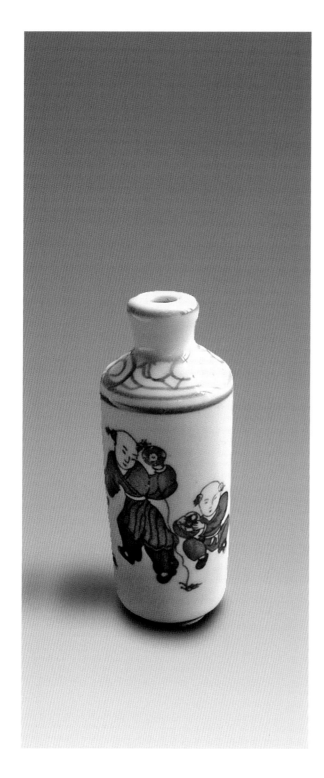

瓷药瓶

近代

瓷质

口径 0.6 厘米，腹宽 3.3 厘米，高 9 厘米

圆柱形，撇口，束颈，溜肩。肩部饰云纹，器身绘两小儿嬉戏图案。青花圆药瓶。

江苏省中医药博物馆藏

Porcelain Medicine Bottle

Modern Times

Porcelain

Mouth Diameter 0.6 cm/ Belly Width 3.3 cm/ Height 9 cm

The column-shaped bottle has a flared mouth, a contracted neck and a smooth shoulder. The shoulder is decorated with cloud patters and the body is painted with the design of two little children playing.

Preserved in Jiangsu Museum of Traditional Chinese Medicine

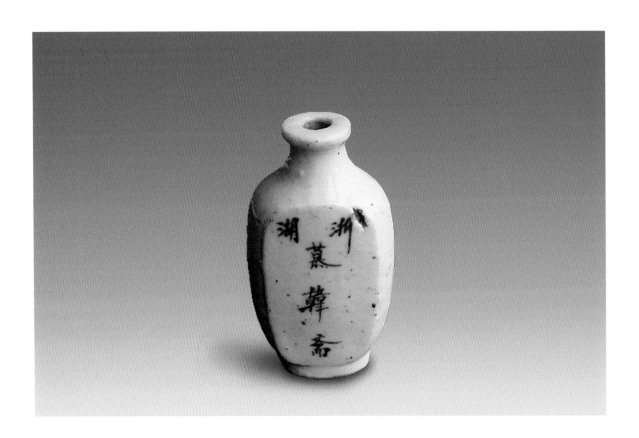

瓷药瓶

近代

瓷质

口径 1 厘米，腹宽 2.4 厘米，高 8.2 厘米

Porcelain Medicine Bottle

Modern Times

Porcelain

Mouth Diameter 1 cm/ Belly Width 2.4 cm/ Height 8.2 cm

撇口，短颈，溜肩，平底。有"浙湖""慕韩斋"

字样。

江苏省中医药博物馆藏

The bottle has a flared mouth, a short neck, a smooth shoulder and a flat bottom. It is inscribed with the Chinese characters "Zhe Hu" and "Mu Han Zhai", meaning the name of the drugstore.

Preserved in Jiangsu Museum of Traditional Chinese Medicine

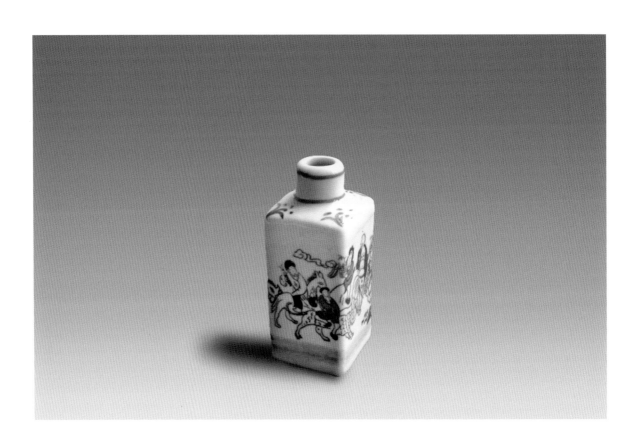

瓷药瓶

近代

瓷质

口径 0.9 厘米，宽 3 厘米，高 7.3 厘米

直口，长颈，溜肩，方柱形，四方底，绘人物图，青花方药瓶。

江苏省中医药博物馆藏

Porcelain Medicine Bottle

Modern Times

Porcelain

Mouth Diameter 0.9 cm/ Width 3 cm/ Height 7.3 cm

The square column bottle has a straight mouth, a long neck, a smooth shoulder and a square bottom. It is painted with figure images.

Preserved in Jiangsu Museum of Traditional Chinese Medicine

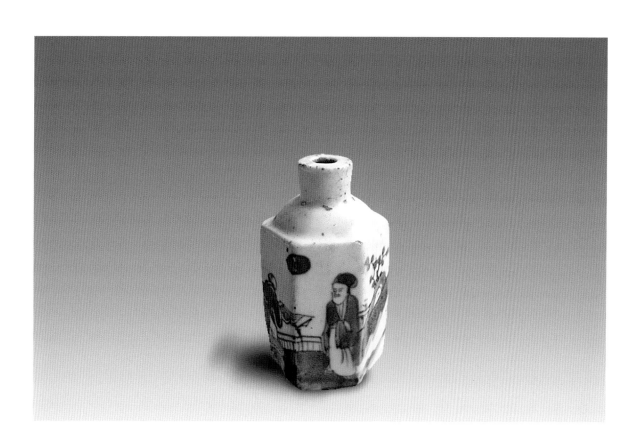

瓷药瓶

近代

瓷质

口径 1 厘米，宽 4 厘米，高 8.2 厘米

直口，长颈，溜肩，瓶腹为六面体，绘青花风景
人物图，平底。

江苏省中医药博物馆藏

Porcelain Medicine Bottle

Modern Times

Porcelain

Mouth Diameter 1 cm/ Belly Width 4 cm/ Height
8.2 cm

The bottle has a straight mouth, a long neck, a
smooth shoulder and a flat bottom. The belly of
the bottle is a hexahedron. It is painted with blue
and white landscapes and figure images.

Preserved in Jiangsu Museum of Traditional

Chinese Medicine

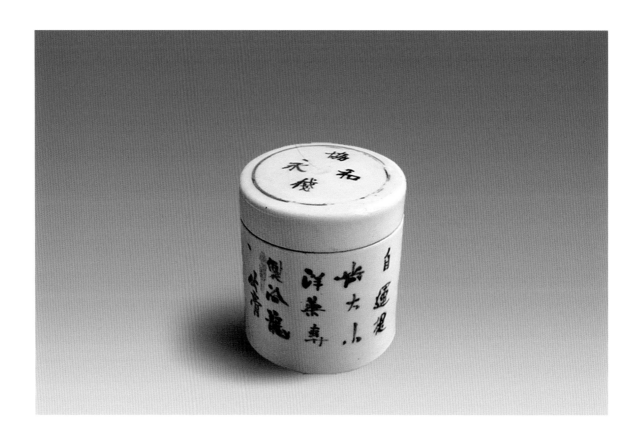

瓷药瓶

近代

瓷质

口径 6.1 厘米，高 8 厘米

圆柱体，有"永和协栈"等字样。

江苏省中医药博物馆藏

Porcelain Medicine Bottle

Modern Times

Porcelain

Mouth Diameter 6.1 cm/ Height 8 cm

The column-shaped bottle is inscribed with the Chinese characters "Yong He Xie Zhan", meaning the name of the drugstore.

Preserved in Jiangsu Museum of Traditional Chinese Medicine

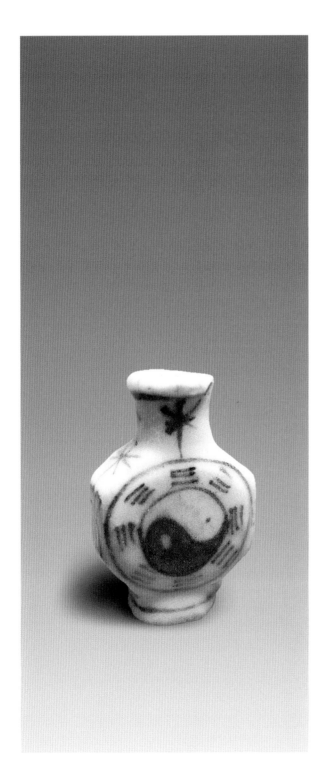

药瓶

近代

瓷质

宽 2.5 厘米，厚 1.2 厘米，高 3.8 厘米

瓶身为八边形，正反两面均为阴阳八卦图。

北京中医药大学中医药博物馆藏

Medicine Bottle

Modern Times

Porcelain

Width 2.5 cm/ Thickness 1.2 cm/ Height 3.8 cm

The bottle is in the shape of an octagon with Eight Diagrams of Yin and Yang on both sides of the bottle.

Preserved in the Museum of Chinese Medicine, Beijing University of Chinese Medicine

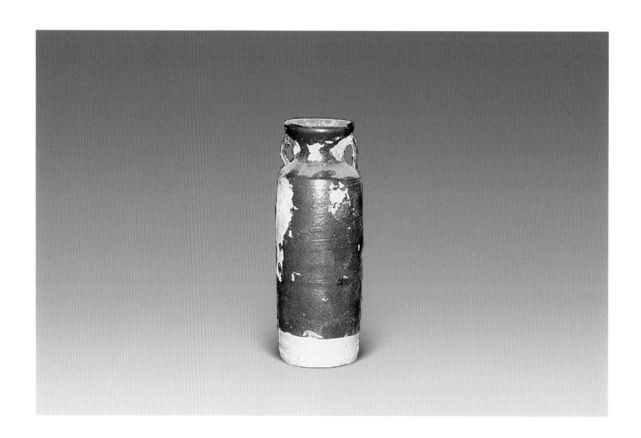

棕釉双耳小药瓶

近代

瓷质

口径 3.8 厘米，底径 4.3 厘米，高 13.3 厘米，重 200 克

Small Brown Glazed Medicine Bottle with Double Handles

Modern Times

Porcelain

Mouth Diameter 3.8 cm/ Bottom Diameter 4.3 cm/ Height 13.3 cm/ Weight 200 g

盘口，短颈，颈肩部有双耳，斜肩，直腹，圈足，腹下部无釉。生活器具，完整。陕西省澄城县征集。

陕西医史博物馆藏

The bottle has a dish-shaped mouth, a short neck, a sloping shoulder, a straight belly, and a ring foot. Between the neck and shoulder are double handles and the lower part of its belly is unglazed. It was utilized as a living utensil and kept intact. It was collected from Chengcheng County, Shaanxi Province.

Preserved in Shaanxi Museum of Medical History

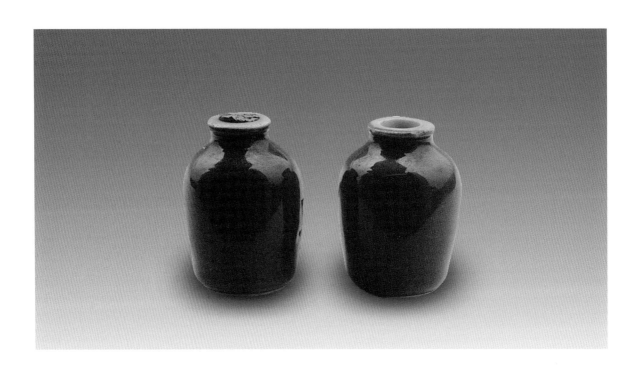

大照康制小药瓶两件

近代

瓷质

左：口外径 3.1 厘米，腹径 4.8 厘米，底径 3.8 厘米，通高 6.4 厘米，重 89 克

右：口外径 2.7 厘米，腹径 4.8 厘米，底径 3.7 厘米，通高 6.2 厘米，重 85.5 克

Small Medicine Bottles Made by Da Zhaokang

Modern Times

Porcelain

The Left Bottle: Mouth Outer Diameter 3.1 cm/ Belly Diameter 4.8 cm/ Bottom Diameter 3.8 cm/ Height 6.4 cm/ Weight 89 g

The Right Bottle: Mouth Outer Diameter 2.7 cm/ Belly Diameter 4.8 cm/ Bottom Diameter 3.7 cm/ Height 6.2 cm/ Weight 85.5 g

撇口，短颈，溜肩，圆圈足，平底。装药用。

广东中医药博物馆藏

The bottles have flared mouths, short necks, smooth shoulders, ring feet and flat bottoms. They were utilized for storing medicine.

Preserved in Guangdong Chinese Medicine Museum

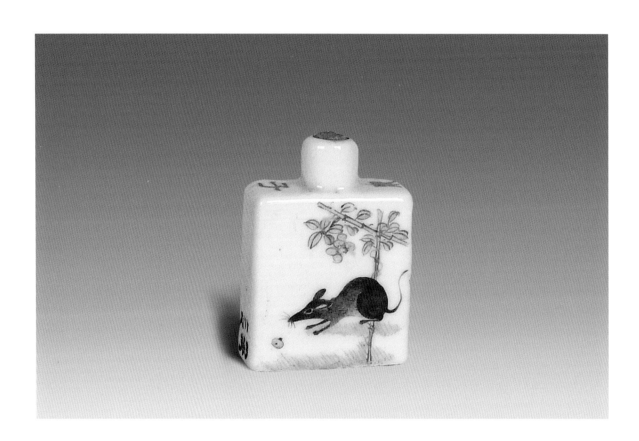

瓷药瓶

民国时期

瓷质

Porcelain Medicine Bottle

Republican Period

Porcelain

扁方形，为盛药器具。该藏品通身以乳白釉为底色，绘粉彩生肖图案，瓷质较细，瓶底有釉无款，瓶肩部颈两端分别有地支名与相应生肖动物名（如子与鼠、申与猴等）字样。此瓶为子鼠瓶，瓶底贴一粉红色纸上写"冰射散"三字，保存基本完好。1957 年入藏。

中华医学会 / 上海中医药博物馆藏

The cuboid bottle was for storing medicine. It is covered with opal glaze on which the animal of Chinese zodiac was painted in famille rose. The quality of the porcelain is fine and smooth. There is no inscription on the glazed base. At each end of its shoulder is inscribed with the names of terrestrial branch and relevant animals such as Zi and Shu (meaning mouse), Shen and Hou (meaning monkey) in zodiac system. The bottle is decorated with designs of Zi Shu (meaning Mouse) with a pink paper writing "Bing She San" attached to the base, meaning the name of the drug. The bottle is still in good condition. It was collected in the year 1957.

Preserved in Chinese Medical Association/ Museum of Chinese Medicine, Shanghai University of Traditional Chinese Medicine

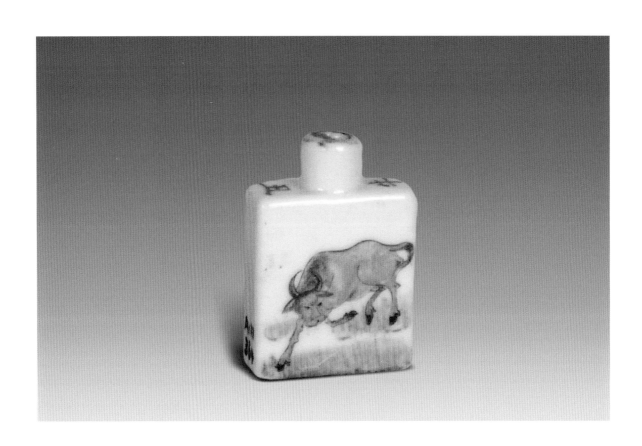

瓷药瓶

民国时期

瓷质

Porcelain Medicine Bottle

Republican Period

Porcelain

扁方形，为盛药器具。该藏品通身以乳白釉为底色，绘粉彩生肖图案，瓷质较细，瓶底有釉无款，瓶肩部颈两端分别有地支名与相应生肖动物名（如子与鼠、申与猴等）字样。此瓶为丑牛瓶，瓶底贴一粉红色纸上写"冰片散"三字，保存基本完好。1957 年入藏。

中华医学会／上海中医药博物馆藏

The cuboid bottle was for storing medicine. It is covered with opal glaze on which the animal of Chinese zodiac was painted in famille rose. The quality of the porcelain is fine and smooth. There is no inscription on the glazed base. At each end of its shoulder is inscribed with the names of terrestrial branch and relevant animals such as Zi and Shu (meaning mouse), Shen and Hou (meaning monkey) in zodiac system. Te bottle is decorated with designs of Chou Niu (meaning bull) with a pink paper writing "Bing Pian San" attached to the base, meaning the name of the drug. The bottle is still in good condition It was collected in the year 1957.
Preserved in Chinese Medical Association/ Museum of Chinese Medicine, Shanghai University of Traditional Chinese Medicine

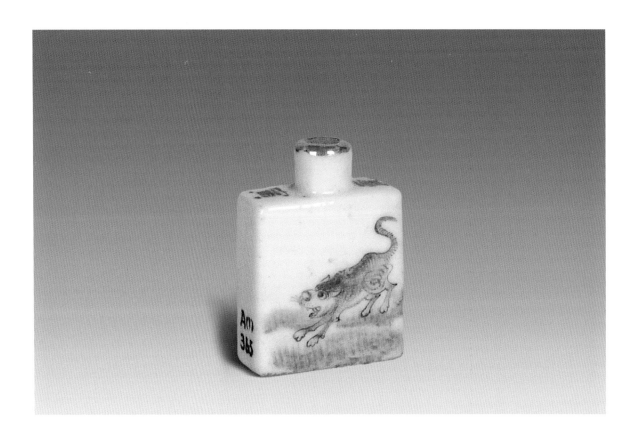

瓷药瓶

民国时期

瓷质

Porcelain Medicine Bottle

Republican Period

Porcelain

扁方形，为盛药器具。该藏品通身以乳白釉为底色，绘粉彩生肖图案，瓷质较细，瓶底有釉无款，瓶肩部颈两端分别有地支名与相应生肖动物名（如子与鼠、申与猴等）字样。此瓶为寅虎瓶，瓶底贴一粉红色纸上写"珠黄"二字，保存基本完好。1957 年入藏。

中华医学会 / 上海中医药博物馆藏

The cuboid bottle for storing medicine. It is covered with opal glaze on which the animal of Chinese zodiac was painted in famille rose. The quality of the porcelain is fine and smooth. There is no inscription on the glazed base. At each end of its shoulder is inscribed with the names of terrestrial branch and relevant animals such as Zi and Shu (meaning mouse)，Shen and Hou (meaning monkey) in zodiac system. The bottle is decorated with the design of Yin Hu (meaning tiger) with a pink paper writing "Zhu Huang" attached to the base, meaning the name of the drug. The bottle is still in good condition It was collected in the year 1957.
Preserved in Chinese Medical Association/ Museum of Chinese Medicine, Shanghai University of Traditional Chinese Medicine

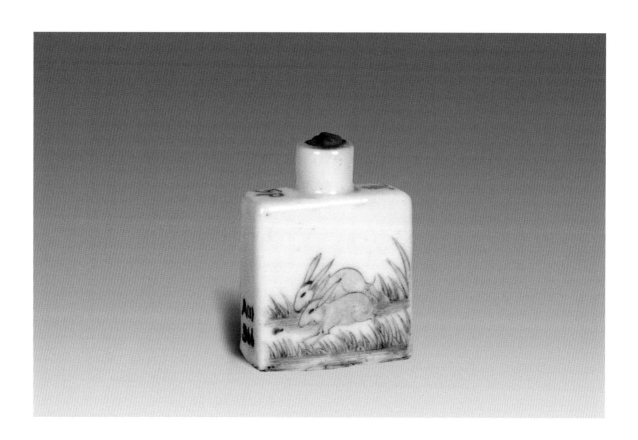

瓷药瓶

民国时期

瓷质

Porcelain Medicine Bottle

Republican Period

Porcelain

扁方形，为盛药器具。该藏品通身以乳白釉为底色，绘粉彩生肖图案，瓷质较细，瓶底有釉无款，瓶肩部颈两端分别有地支名与相应生肖动物名（如子与鼠、申与猴等）字样。此瓶为卯兔瓶，瓶底贴一粉红色纸上写"冰硼散"三字，保存基本完好。1957年入藏。

中华医学会／上海中医药博物馆藏

The cuboid bottle was for storing medicine. It is covered with opal glaze on which the animal of Chinese zodiac was painted in famille rose. The quality of the porcelain is fine and smooth. There is no inscription on the glazed base. At each end of its shoulder is inscribed with the names of terrestrial branch and relevant animals such as Zi and Shu (meaning mouse), Shen and Hou (meaning monkey) in zodiac system. The bottle is decorated with the designs of Mao Tu (meaning rabbit) with a pink paper writing "Bing Peng San" attached to the base, meaning the name of the drug. The bottle is still in good condition was collected in the year 1957.

Preserved in Chinese Medical Association/ Museum of Chinese Medicine, Shanghai University of Traditional Chinese Medicine

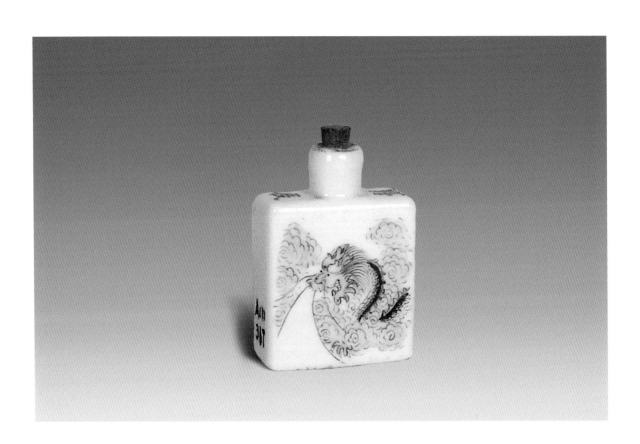

瓷药瓶

民国时期

瓷质

Porcelain Medicine Bottle

Republican Period

Porcelain

扁方形，为盛药器具。该藏品通身以乳白釉为
底色，绘粉彩生肖图案，瓷质较细，瓶底有釉
无款，瓶肩部颈两端分别有地支名与相应生肖
动物名（如子与鼠、申与猴等）字样。此瓶为
辰龙瓶，瓶底贴一粉红色纸上写"红雪"二字，
保存基本完好。1957 年入藏。

中华医学会 / 上海中医药博物馆藏

The cuboid bottle was for storing medicine. It
is covered with opal glaze on which the animal
of Chinese zodiac was painted in famille rose.
The quality of the porcelain is fine and smooth.
There is no inscription on the glazed base. At
each end of its shoulder is inscribed with the
names of terrestrial branch and relevant animals
such as Zi and Shu (meaning mouse)，Shen
and Hou (meaning monkey) in zodiac system.
The bottle is decorated with the designs of Chen
Long (meaning dragon) with a pink paper writing
"Hong Xue" attached to the base, meaning the
name of the drug. The bottle is still in good
condition It was collected in the year 1957.
Preserved in Chinese Medical Association/
Museum of Chinese Medicine, Shanghai
University of Traditional Chinese Medicine

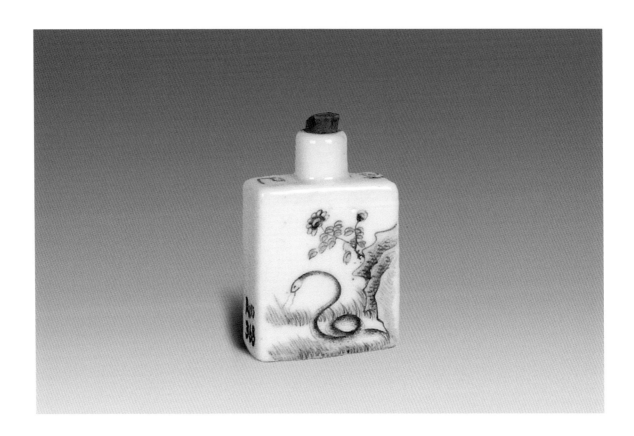

瓷药瓶

民国时期

瓷质

Porcelain Medicine Bottle

Republican Period

Porcelain

扁方形，为盛药器具。该藏品通身以乳白釉为底色，绘粉彩生肖图案，瓷质较细，瓶底有釉无款，瓶肩部颈两端分别有地支名与相应生肖动物名（如子与鼠、申与猴等）字样。此瓶为巳蛇瓶，瓶底贴一粉红色纸上写"黄雪"二字，保存基本完好。1957 年入藏。

中华医学会 / 上海中医药博物馆藏

The cuboid bottle was for storing medicine. It is covered with opal glaze on which the animal of Chinese zodiac was painted in famille rose. The quality of the porcelain is fine and smooth. There is no inscription on the glazed base. At each end of its shoulder is inscribed with the names of terrestrial branch and relevant animals such as Zi and Shu (meaning mouse), Shen and Hou (meaning monkey) in zodiac system. The bottle is decorated with the designs of Si She (meaning snake) with a pink paper writing "Huang Xue" attached to the base, meaning the name of the drug. The bottle is still in good condition It was collected in the year 1957.

Preserved in Chinese Medical Association/ Museum of Chinese Medicine, Shanghai University of Traditional Chinese Medicine

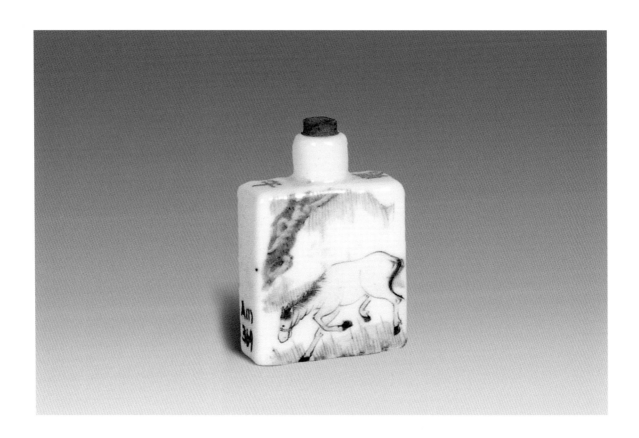

瓷药瓶

民国时期

瓷质

Porcelain Medicine Bottle

Republican Period

Porcelain

扁方形，为盛药器具。该藏品通身以乳白釉为底色，绘粉彩生肖图案，瓷质较细，瓶底有釉无款，瓶肩部颈两端分别有地支名与相应生肖动物名（如子与鼠、申与猴等）字样。此瓶为午马瓶，瓶底贴一粉红色纸上写"碧雪"二字，保存基本完好。1957 年入藏。

中华医学会 / 上海中医药博物馆藏

The cuboid bottle was for storing medicine. It is covered with opal glaze on which the animal of Chinese zodiac was painted in famille rose. The quality of the porcelain is fine and smooth. There is no inscription on the glazed base. At each end of its shoulder is inscribed with the names of terrestrial branch and relevant animals such as Zi and Shu (meaning mouse), Shen and Hou (meaning monkey) in zodiac system. The bottle is decorated with the designs of Wu Ma (meaning horse) with a pink paper writing "Bi Xue" attached to the base, meaning the name of the drug. The bottle is still in good condition It was collected in the year 1957.

Preserved in Chinese Medical Association/ Museum of Chinese Medicine, Shanghai University of Traditional Chinese Medicine

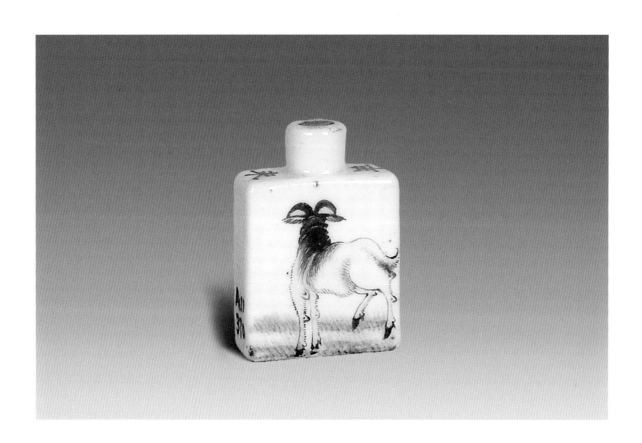

瓷药瓶

民国时期

瓷质

Porcelain Medicine Bottle

Republican Period

Porcelain

扁方形，为盛药器具。该藏品通身以乳白釉为底色，绘粉彩生肖图案，瓷质较细，瓶底有釉无款，瓶肩部颈两端分别有地支名与相应生肖动物名（如子与鼠、申与猴等）字样。此瓶为未羊瓶，瓶底贴一粉红色纸上写"五宝"二字，保存基本完好。1957 年入藏。

中华医学会 / 上海中医药博物馆藏

The cuboid bottle was for storing medicine. It is covered with opal glaze on which the animal of Chinese zodiac was painted in famille rose. The quality of the porcelain is fine and smooth. There is no inscription on the glazed base. At each end of its shoulder is inscribed with the names of terrestrial branch and relevant animals such as Zi and Shu (meaning mouse), Shen and Hou (meaning monkey) in zodiac system. The bottle is decorated with the designs of Wei Yang (meaning goat) with a pink paper writing "Wu Bao" attached to the base, meaning the name of the drug. The bottle is still in good condition It was collected in the year 1957.

Preserved in Chinese Medical Association/ Museum of Chinese Medicine, Shanghai University of Traditional Chinese Medicine

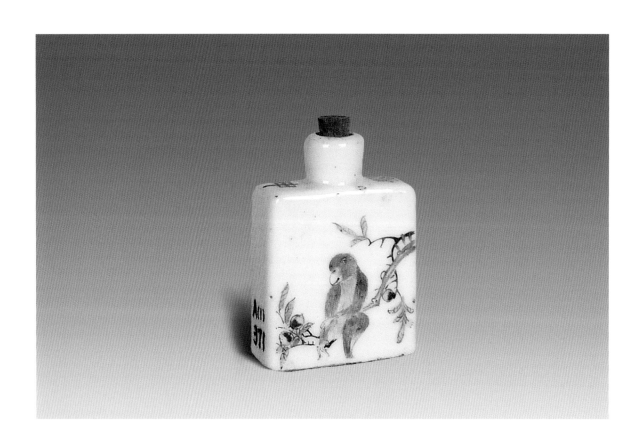

瓷药瓶

民国时期

瓷质

Porcelain Medicine Bottle

Republican Period

Porcelain

扁方形，为盛药器具。该藏品通身以乳白釉为
底色，绘粉彩生肖图案，瓷质较细，瓶底有釉
无款，瓶肩部颈两端分别有地支名与相应生肖
动物名（如子与鼠、申与猴等）字样。此瓶为
申猴瓶，瓶底贴一粉红色纸上写"如意"二字，
保存基本完好。1957 年入藏。

中华医学会 / 上海中医药博物馆藏

The cuboid bottle was for storing medicine. It
is covered with opal glaze on which the animal
of Chinese zodiac was painted in famille rose.
The quality of the porcelain is fine and smooth.
There is no inscription on the glazed base. At
each end of its shoulder is inscribed with the
names of terrestrial branch and relevant animals
such as Zi and Shu (meaning mouse), Shen and
Hou (meaning monkey)in zodiac system. The
bottle is decorated with the designs of Shen Hou
(meaning monkey) with a pink paper writing "Ru
Yi" attached to the base, meaning the name of the
drug. The bottle is still in good condition It was
collected in the year 1957.

Preserved in Chinese Medical Association/
Museum of Chinese Medicine, Shanghai
University of Traditional Chinese Medicine

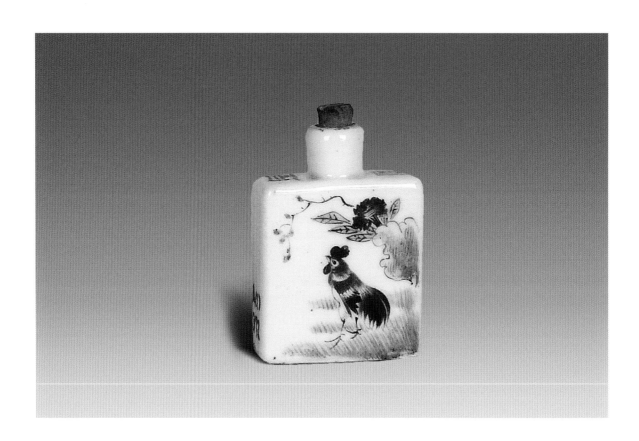

瓷药瓶

民国时期

瓷质

Porcelain Medicine Bottle

Republican Period

Porcelain

扁方形，为盛药器具。该藏品通身以乳白釉为底色，绘粉彩生肖图案，瓷质较细，瓶底有釉无款，瓶肩部颈两端分别有地支名与相应生肖动物名（如子与鼠、申与猴等）字样。此瓶为酉鸡瓶，瓶底贴一粉红色纸上写"金匙"二字，保存基本完好。1957 年入藏。

中华医学会 / 上海中医药博物馆藏

The cuboid bottle was for storing medicine. It is covered with opal glaze on which the animal of Chinese zodiac was painted in famille rose. The quality of the porcelain is fine and smooth. There is no inscription on the glazed base. At each end of its shoulder is inscribed with the names of terrestrial branch and relevant animals such as Zi and Shu (meaning mouse)，Shen and Hou (meaning monkey) in zodiac system. The bottle is decorated with the designs of You Ji (meaning rooster) with a pink paper writing "Jin Shi" attached to the base, meaning the name of the drug. The bottle is still in good condition It was collected in the year 1957. Preserved in Chinese Medical Association/ Museum of Chinese Medicine, Shanghai University of Traditional Chinese Medicine

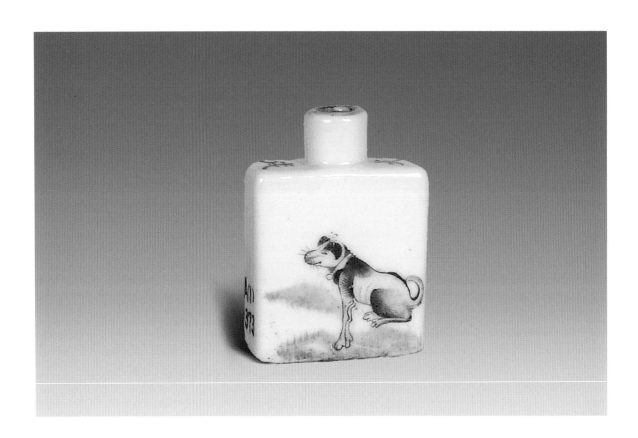

瓷药瓶

民国时期

瓷质

Porcelain Medicine Bottle

Republican Period

Porcelain

扁方形，为盛药器具。该藏品通身以乳白釉为底色，绘粉彩生肖图案，瓷质较细，瓶底有釉无款，瓶肩部颈两端分别有地支名与相应生肖动物名（如子与鼠、申与猴等）字样。此瓶为戌狗瓶，瓶底贴一粉红色纸上写"玉匙"二字，保存基本完好。1957 年入藏。

中华医学会 / 上海中医药博物馆藏

The cuboid bottle was for storing medicine. It is covered with opal glaze on which the animal of Chinese zodiac was painted in famille rose. The quality of the porcelain is fine and smooth. There is no inscription on the glazed base. At each end of its shoulder is inscribed with the names of terrestrial branch and relevant animals such as Zi and Shu (meaning mouse), Shen and Hou (meaning monkey) in zodiac system. The bottle is decorated with the designs of Xu Gou (meaning dog) with a pink paper writing "Yu Shi" attached to the base, meaning the name of the drug. The bottle is still in good condition It was collected in the year 1957.

Preserved in Chinese Medical Association/ Museum of Chinese Medicine, Shanghai University of Traditional Chinese Medicine

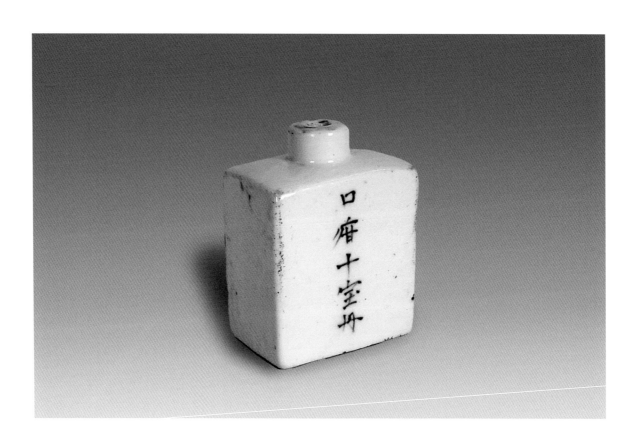

瓷药瓶

民国时期

瓷质

宽 7.1 厘米，厚 4.8 厘米，通高 9 厘米

Porcelain Medicine Bottle

Republican Period

Porcelain

Width 7.1 cm/ Thickness 4.8 cm/ Height 9 cm

扁方形，通身施乳白釉，瓷质较粗糙，瓶底无釉呈棕黑色，瓶身烧蓝字"口疳十宝丹"。盛药器具。保存基本完好。

中华医学会 / 上海中医药博物馆藏

The cuboid bottle was for storing medicine. It is covered with opal glaze. The bottom is unglazed, brown and black; the body is painted with blue Chinese characters "Kou Gan Shi Bao Dan", meaning the name of the drug. The quality of the porcelain is rough. It is still in good condition.

Preserved in Chinese Medical Association/ Museum of Chinese Medicine, Shanghai University of Traditional Chinese Medicine

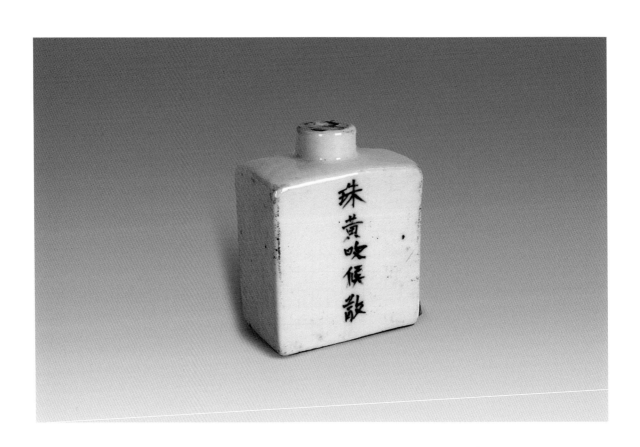

瓷药瓶

民国时期

瓷质

宽 7.1 厘米，厚 4.8 厘米，通高 9 厘米

Porcelain Medicine Bottle

Republican Period

Porcelain

Width 7.1 cm/ Thickness 4.8 cm/ Height 9 cm

扁方形，通身施乳白釉，表面较粗糙，瓶
底未施釉呈棕黑色，瓶身烧蓝字"珠黄吹
喉散"。盛药器具。保存基本完好。

中华医学会 / 上海中医药博物馆藏

The cuboid bottle was for storing medicine.
It is covered with opal glaze. The bottom is
brownish black and unglazed; the body is
painted with blue Chinese characters "Zhu
Huang Chui Hou San", meaning the name
of the drug. The quality of the porcelain is
rough. It is still in good condition.
Preserved in Chinese Medical Association/
Museum of Chinese Medicine, Shanghai
University of Traditional Chinese Medicine

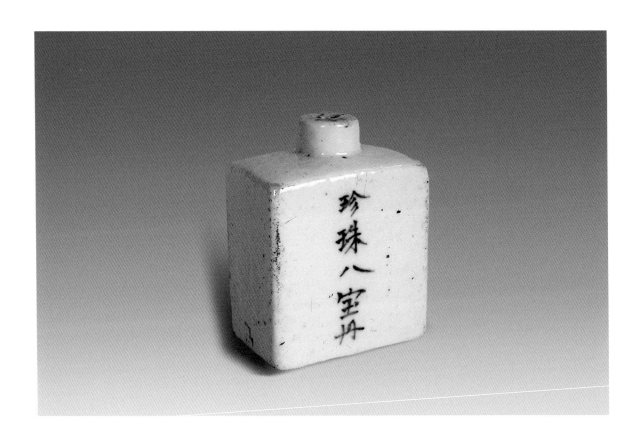

瓷药瓶

民国时期

瓷质

宽 7.1 厘米，厚 4.8 厘米，通高 9 厘米

Porcelain Medicine Bottle

Republican Period

Porcelain

Width 7.1 cm/ Thickness 4.8 cm/ Height 9 cm

扁方形，通身施乳白釉，表面较粗糙，瓶底未施釉呈棕黑色，瓶身烧蓝字"珍珠八宝丹"。盛药器具。保存基本完好。

中华医学会 / 上海中医药博物馆藏

The cuboid bottle was for storing medicine. It is covered with opal glaze. The bottom is brownish black and unglazed; the body is painted with blue Chinese characters "Zhen Zhu Ba Bao Dan", meaning the name of the drug. The quality of the porcelain is rough. It is still in good condition.

Preserved in Chinese Medical Association/ Museum of Chinese Medicine, Shanghai University of Traditional Chinese Medicine

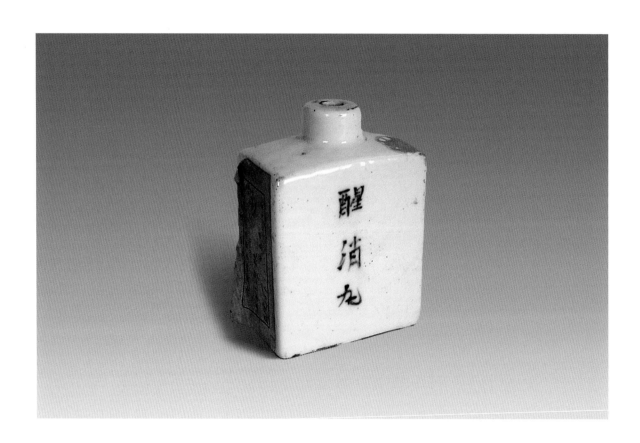

瓷药瓶

民国时期

瓷质

宽 7.1 厘米，厚 4.8 厘米，通高 9 厘米

Porcelain Medicine Bottle

Republican Period

Porcelain

Width 7.1 cm/ Thickness 4.8 cm/ Height 9 cm

扁方形，通身施乳白釉，表面较粗糙，瓶
底未施釉呈棕黑色，瓶身烧蓝字"醒消丸"。
盛药器具。保存基本完好。

中华医学会 / 上海中医药博物馆藏

The cuboid bottle was for storing medicine.
It is covered with opal glaze. The bottom is
brownish black and unglazed; the body is
painted with blue Chinese characters "Xing
Xiao Wan", meaning the name of the drug.
The quality of the porcelain is rough. It is
still in good condition.
Preserved in Chinese Medical Association/
Museum of Chinese Medicine, Shanghai
University of Traditional Chinese Medicine

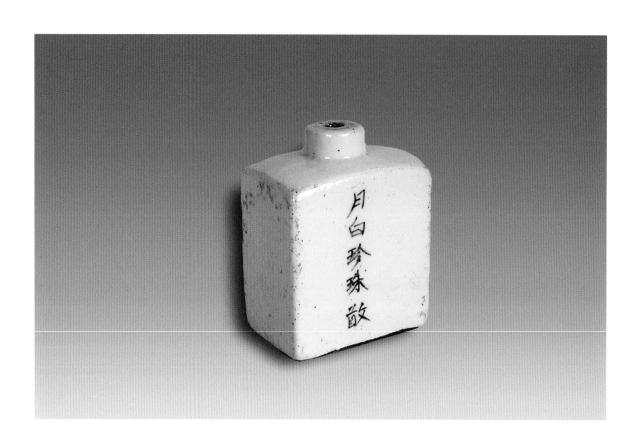

瓷药瓶

民国时期

瓷质

宽 7.1 厘米，厚 4.8 厘米，通高 9 厘米

Porcelain Medicine Bottle

Republican Period

Porcelain

Width 7.1 cm/ Thickness 4.8 cm/ Height 9 cm

扁方形，通身施乳白釉，表面较粗糙，瓶
底未施釉呈棕黑色，瓶身烧蓝字"月白珍
珠散"。盛药器具。保存基本完好。

中华医学会 / 上海中医药博物馆藏

The cuboid bottle was for storing medicine.
It is covered with opal glaze. The bottom is
brownish black and unglazed; the body is
painted with blue Chinese characters "Yue
Bai Zhen Zhu San", meaning the name of
the drug. The quality of the porcelain is
rough. It is still in good condition.
Preserved in Chinese Medical Association/
Museum of Chinese Medicine, Shanghai
University of Traditional Chinese Medicine

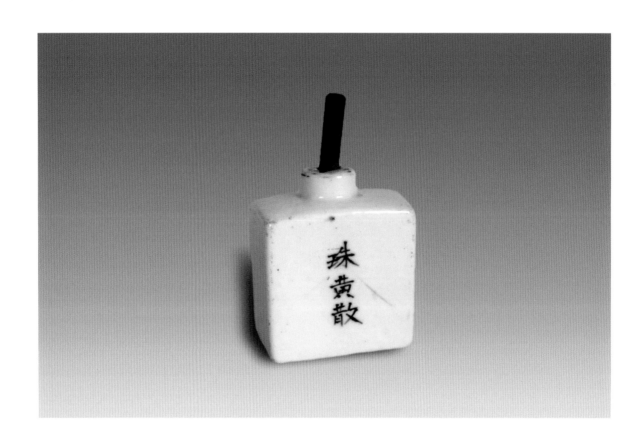

瓷药瓶

民国时期

瓷质

宽 7.1 厘米，厚 4.8 厘米，通高 9 厘米

Porcelain Medicine Bottle

Republican Period

Porcelain

Width 7.1 cm/ Thickness 4.8 cm/ Height 9 cm

扁方形，通身施乳白釉，表面较粗糙，瓶
底未施釉呈棕黑色，瓶身烧蓝字"珠黄散"。
盛药器具。保存基本完好。

中华医学会 / 上海中医药博物馆藏

The cuboid bottle was for storing medicine.
It is covered with opal glaze. The bottom is
brownish black and unglazed; the body is
painted with blue Chinese characters "Zhu
Huang San", meaning the name of the
drug. The quality of the porcelain is rough.
It is still in good condition.

Preserved in Chinese Medical Association/
Museum of Chinese Medicine, Shanghai
University of Traditional Chinese Medicine

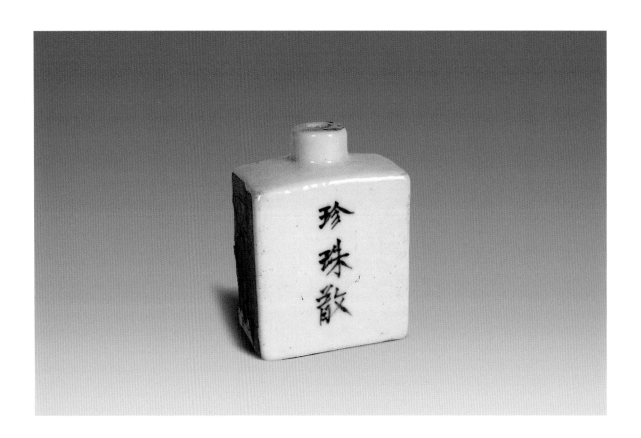

瓷药瓶

民国时期

瓷质

宽 7.1 厘米，厚 4.8 厘米，通高 9 厘米

Porcelain Medicine Bottle

Republican Period

Porcelain

Width 7.1 cm/ Thickness 4.8 cm/ Height 9 cm

扁瓶状，通身施乳白釉，瓷质较粗糙，瓶底无釉呈棕黑色，瓶身烧蓝字"珍珠散"。盛药器具。保存基本完好。1955 年入藏。

中华医学会 / 上海中医药博物馆藏

The cuboid bottle was for storing medicine. It is covered with opal glaze. The bottom is brownish black and unglazed; the body is painted with blue Chinese characters "Zhen Zhu San", meaning the name of the drug. The quality of the porcelain is rough. The bottle is still in good condition It was collected in the year 1955.

Preserved in Chinese Medical Association/ Museum of Chinese Medicine, Shanghai University of Traditional Chinese Medicine

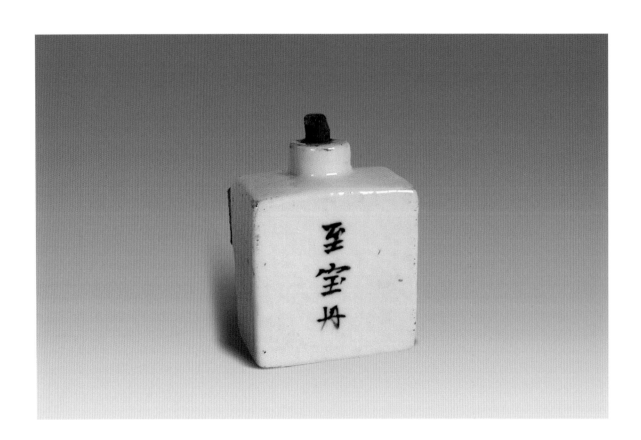

瓷药瓶

近现代

瓷质

宽 7.1 厘米，厚 4.8 厘米，通高 9 厘米

Porcelain Medicine Bottle

Modern Times

Porcelain

Width 7.1 cm/ Thickness 4.8 cm/ Height 9 cm

扁瓶状，通身施乳白釉，瓷质较粗糙，瓶底无釉呈棕黑色，瓶身烧蓝字"至宝丹"。盛药器具。保存基本完好。1955年入藏。

中华医学会 / 上海中医药博物馆藏

The cuboid bottle was for storing medicine. It is covered with opal glaze. The bottom is brownish black and unglazed; the body is painted with blue Chinese characters as "Zhi Bao Dan", meaning the name of the drug. The quality of the porcelain is rough. The bottle is still in good condition It was collected in the year 1955.

Preserved in Chinese Medical Association/ Museum of Chinese Medicine, Shanghai University of Traditional Chinese Medicine

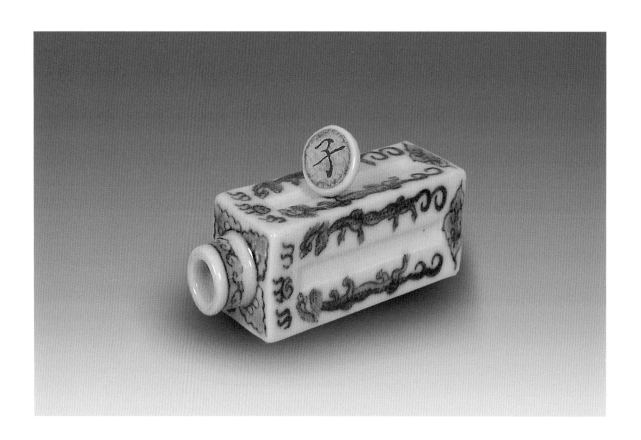

药瓶

近现代

瓷质

边长 2.6 厘米，通高 8.6 厘米

Medicine Bottle

Modern Times

Porcelain

Side Length 2.6 cm/ Height 8.6 cm

方瓶形，盛药器具。该藏品为我馆收藏的
南翔张志方中药室红木药箱内配瓷药瓶之
一，青花瓷，双龙戏珠纹，平底直口，上
配瓷瓶盖，每个瓶盖上粘有药名标签，做
工精细，造型美观，保存基本完好。1959
年入藏。

中华医学会 / 上海中医药博物馆藏

The square bottle was for storing medicine.
It is one of the porcelain medicine bottles
equipped in the mahogany medicine chest
in Zhang Zhifang Traditional Chinese
Medicine Store at Nanxiang. The blue and
white porcelain bottle is decorated with the
design of two dragons playing a fireball.
It has a flat bottom and a straight mouth
and each porcelain cover is pasted a tag of
medicine name. Its craft is exquisite and
elegant. The bottle is still in good condition.
It was collected in the year 1959.
Preserved in Chinese Medical Association/
Museum of Chinese Medicine, Shanghai
University of Traditional Chinese Medicine

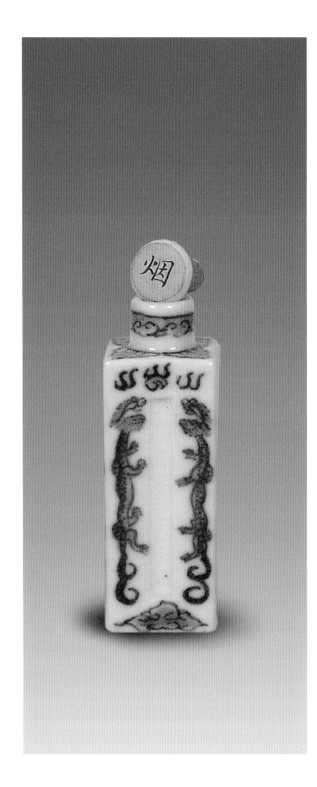

药瓶

近现代

瓷质

边长 2.6 厘米，通高 8.6 厘米

Medicine Bottle

Modern Times

Porcelain

Side Length 2.6 cm/ Height 8.6 cm

方瓶形，盛药器具。该藏品为我馆收藏的
南翔张志方中药室红木药箱内配瓷药瓶之
一，青花瓷，双龙戏珠纹，平底直口，上
配瓷瓶盖，每个瓶盖上粘有药名标签，做
工精细，造型美观，保存基本完好。1959
年入藏。

中华医学会 / 上海中医药博物馆藏

The bottle is square for storing medicine.
It is one of the porcelain medicine bottles
equipped in the mahogany medicine chest
in Zhang Zhifang Traditional Chinese
Medicine Store at Nanxiang. The blue and
white porcelain bottle is decorated with the
design of two dragons playing a fireball.
It has a flat bottom and a straight mouth
and each porcelain cover is pasted a tag of
medicine name. Its craft is exquisite and
elegant. It is still in good condition and
was collected in the year 1959.
Preserved in Chinese Medical Association/
Museum of Chinese Medicine, Shanghai
University of Traditional Chinese Medicine

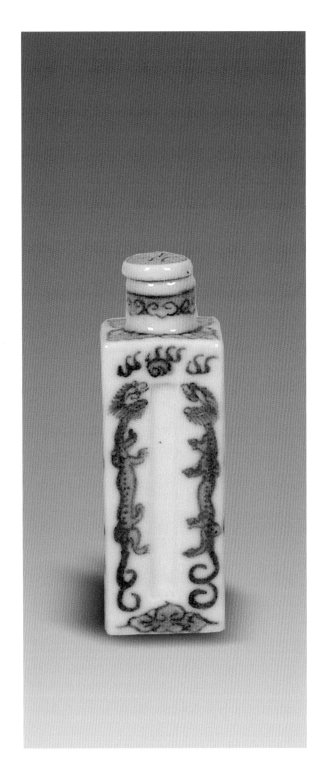

药瓶

近现代

瓷质

长 2.6 厘米，通高 8.6 厘米

Medicine Bottle

Modern Times

Porcelain

Side length 2.6 cm/ Height 8.6 cm

方瓶形，盛药器具。该藏品为我馆收藏的
南翔张志方中药室红木药箱内配瓷药瓶之
一，青花瓷，双龙戏珠纹，平底直口，上
配瓷瓶盖，每个瓶盖上粘有药名标签，做
工精细，造型美观，保存基本完好。1959
年入藏。

中华医学会／上海中医药博物馆藏

The bottle is square for storing medicine.
It is one of the porcelain medicine bottles
equipped in the mahogany medicine chest
in Zhang Zhifang Traditional Chinese
Medicine Store at Nanxiang. The blue and
white porcelain bottle is decorated with the
design of two dragons playing a fireball.
It has a flat bottom and a straight mouth
and each porcelain cover is pasted a tag of
medicine name. Its craft is exquisite and
elegant. It is still in good condition. and was
collected in the year 1959.

Preserved in Chinese Medical Association/
Museum of Chinese Medicine, Shanghai
University of Traditional Chinese Medicine

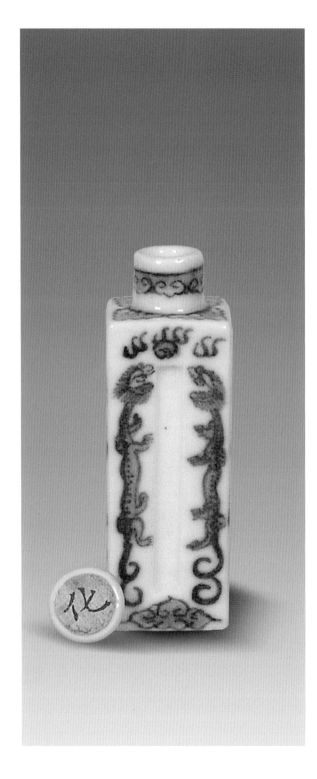

药瓶

近现代

瓷质

边长 2.6 厘米，通高 8.6 厘米

Medicine Bottle

Modern Times

Porcelain

Side Length 2.6 cm/ Height 8.6 cm

方瓶形，盛药器具。该藏品为我馆收藏的
南翔张志方中药室红木药箱内配瓷药瓶之
一，青花瓷，双龙戏珠纹，平底直口，上
配瓷瓶盖，每个瓶盖上粘有药名标签，做
工精细，造型美观，保存基本完好。1959
年入藏。

中华医学会 / 上海中医药博物馆藏

The square bottle was for storing medicine.
It is one of the porcelain medicine bottles
equipped in the mahogany medicine chest
in Zhang Zhifang Traditional Chinese
Medicine Store at Nanxiang. The blue and
white porcelain bottle is decorated with the
design of two dragons playing a fireball.
It has a flat bottom and a straight mouth
and each porcelain cover is pasted a tag of
medicine name. Its craft is exquisite and
elegant. The bottle is still in good condition.
It was collected in the year 1959.
Preserved in Chinese Medical Association/
Museum of Chinese Medicine, Shanghai
University of Traditional Chinese Medicine

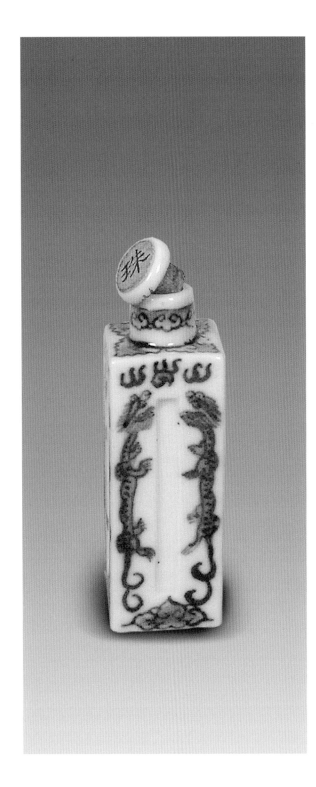

药瓶

近现代

瓷质

边长 2.6 厘米，通高 8.6 厘米

Medicine Bottle

Modern Times

Porcelain

Side Length 2.6 cm/ Height 8.6 cm

方瓶形，盛药器具。该藏品为我馆收藏的南翔张志方中药室红木药箱内配瓷药瓶之一，青花瓷，双龙戏珠纹，平底直口，上配瓷瓶盖，每个瓶盖上粘有药名标签，做工精细，造型美观，保存基本完好。1959年入藏。

中华医学会 / 上海中医药博物馆藏

The square bottle was for storing medicine. It is one of the porcelain medicine bottles equipped in the mahogany medicine chest in Zhang Zhifang Traditional Chinese Medicine Store at Nanxiang. The blue and white porcelain bottle is decorated with the design of two dragons playing a fireball. It has a flat bottom and a straight mouth and each porcelain cover is pasted a tag of medicine name. Its craft is exquisite and elegant. The bottle is still in good condition. It was collected in the year 1959.
Preserved in Chinese Medical Association/ Museum of Chinese Medicine, Shanghai University of Traditional Chinese Medicine

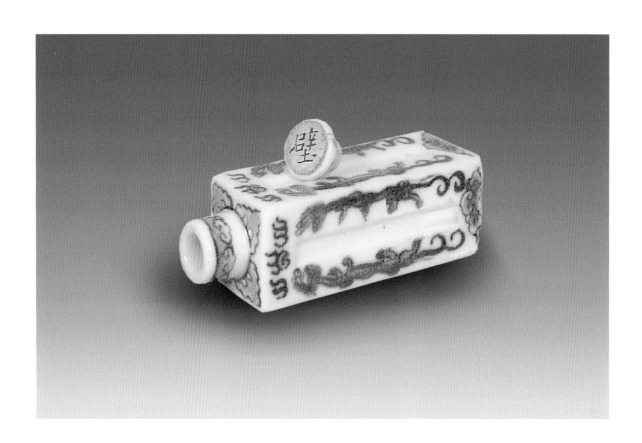

药瓶

近现代

瓷质

边长 2.6 厘米，通高 8.6 厘米

Medicine Bottle

Modern Times

Porcelain

Side Length 2.6 cm/ Height 8.6 cm

方瓶形，盛药器具。该藏品为我馆收藏的南翔张志方中药室红木药箱内配瓷药瓶之一，青花瓷，双龙戏珠纹，平底直口，上配瓷瓶盖，每个瓶盖上粘有药名标签，做工精细，造型美观，保存基本完好。1959年入藏。

中华医学会／上海中医药博物馆藏

The square bottle was for storing medicine. It is one of the porcelain medicine bottles equipped in the mahogany medicine chest in Zhang Zhifang Traditional Chinese Medicine Store at Nanxiang. The blue and white porcelain bottle is decorated with the design of two dragons playing a fireball. It has a flat bottom and a straight mouth and each porcelain cover is pasted a tag of medicine name. Its craft is exquisite and elegant. The bottle is still in good condition. It was collected in the year 1959.

Preserved in Chinese Medical Association/ Museum of Chinese Medicine, Shanghai University of Traditional Chinese Medicine

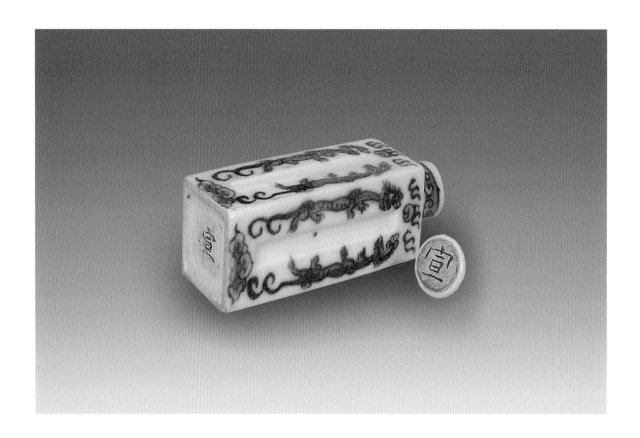

药瓶

近现代

瓷质

边长 2.6 厘米，通高 8.6 厘米

Medicine Bottle

Modern Times

Porcelain

Side Length 2.6 cm/ Height 8.6 cm

方瓶形，盛药器具。该藏品为我馆收藏的南翔张志方中药室红木药箱内配瓷药瓶之一，青花瓷，双龙戏珠纹，平底直口，上配瓷瓶盖，每个瓶盖上粘有药名标签，做工精细，造型美观，保存基本完好。1959年入藏。

中华医学会 / 上海中医药博物馆藏

The square bottle was for storing medicine. It is one of the porcelain medicine bottles equipped in the mahogany medicine chest in Zhang Zhifang Traditional Chinese Medicine Store at Nanxiang. The blue and white porcelain bottle is decorated with the design of two dragons playing a fireball. It has a flat bottom and a straight mouth and each porcelain cover is pasted a tag of medicine name. Its craft is exquisite and elegant. The bottle is still in good condition. It was collected in the year 1959.

Preserved in Chinese Medical Association/ Museum of Chinese Medicine, Shanghai University of Traditional Chinese Medicine

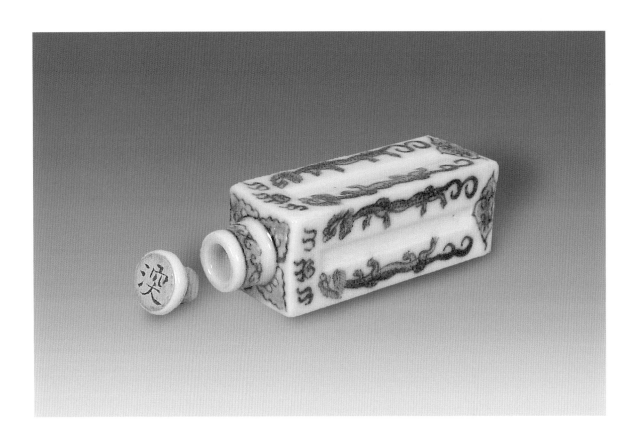

药瓶

近现代

瓷质

边长 2.6 厘米，通高 8.6 厘米

Medicine Bottle

Modern Times

Porcelain

Side Length 2.6 cm/ Height 8.6 cm

方瓶形，盛药器具。该藏品为我馆收藏的南翔张志方中药室红木药箱内配瓷药瓶之一，青花瓷，双龙戏珠纹，平底直口，上配瓷瓶盖，每个瓶盖上粘有药名标签，做工精细，造型美观，保存基本完好。1959年入藏。

中华医学会/上海中医药博物馆藏

The square bottle was for storing medicine. It is one of the porcelain medicine bottles equipped in the mahogany medicine chest in Zhang Zhifang Traditional Chinese Medicine Store at Nanxiang. The blue and white porcelain bottle is decorated with the design of two dragons playing a fireball. It has a flat bottom and a straight mouth and each porcelain cover is pasted a tag of medicine name. Its craft is exquisite and elegant. The bottle is still in good condition. It was collected in the year 1959.

Preserved in Chinese Medical Association/ Museum of Chinese Medicine, Shanghai University of Traditional Chinese Medicine

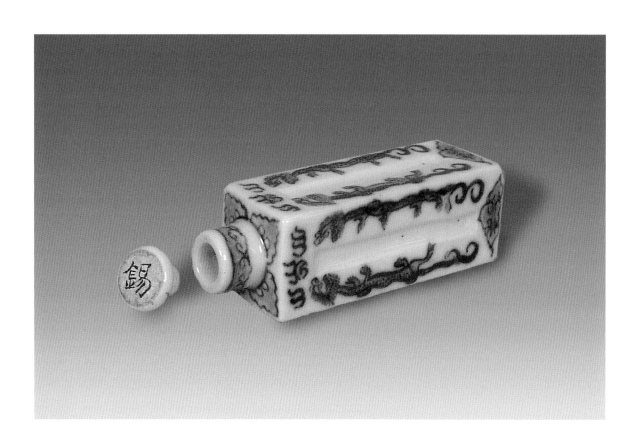

药瓶

近现代

瓷质

边长 2.6 厘米，通高 8.6 厘米

Medicine Bottle

Modern Times

Porcelain

Side length 2.6 cm/ Height 8.6 cm

方瓶形，盛药器具。该藏品为我馆收藏的南翔张志方中药室红木药箱内配瓷药瓶之一，青花瓷，双龙戏珠纹，平底直口，上配瓷瓶盖，每个瓶盖上粘有药名标签，做工精细，造型美观，保存基本完好。1959年入藏。

中华医学会 / 上海中医药博物馆藏

The square bottle was for storing medicine. It is one of the porcelain medicine bottles equipped in the mahogany medicine chest in Zhang Zhifang Traditional Chinese Medicine Store at Nanxiang. The blue and white porcelain bottle is decorated with the design of two dragons playing a fireball. It has a flat bottom and a straight mouth and each porcelain cover is pasted a tag of medicine name. Its craft is exquisite and elegant. The bottle is still in good condition. It was collected in the year 1959.

Preserved in Chinese Medical Association/ Museum of Chinese Medicine, Shanghai University of Traditional Chinese Medicine

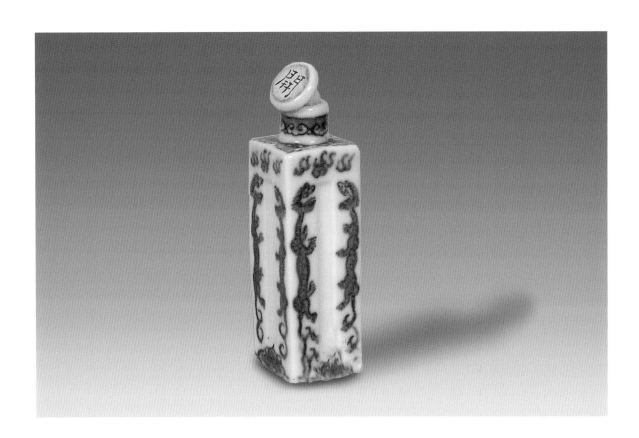

药瓶

近现代

瓷质

边长 2.6 厘米，通高 8.6 厘米

Medicine Bottle

Modern Times

Porcelain

Side Length 2.6 cm/ Height 8.6 cm

方瓶形，盛药器具。该藏品为我馆收藏的南翔张志方中药室红木药箱内配瓷药瓶之一，青花瓷，双龙戏珠纹，平底直口，上配瓷瓶盖，每个瓶盖上粘有药名标签，做工精细，造型美观，保存基本完好。1959年入藏。

中华医学会 / 上海中医药博物馆藏

The square bottle was for storing medicine. It is one of the porcelain medicine bottles equipped in the mahogany medicine chest in Zhang Zhifang Traditional Chinese Medicine Store at Nanxiang. The blue and white porcelain bottle is decorated with the design of two dragons playing a fireball. It has a flat bottom and a straight mouth and each porcelain cover is pasted a tag of medicine name. Its craft is exquisite and elegant. The bottle is still in good condition. It was collected in the year 1959.

Preserved in Chinese Medical Association/ Museum of Chinese Medicine, Shanghai University of Traditional Chinese Medicine

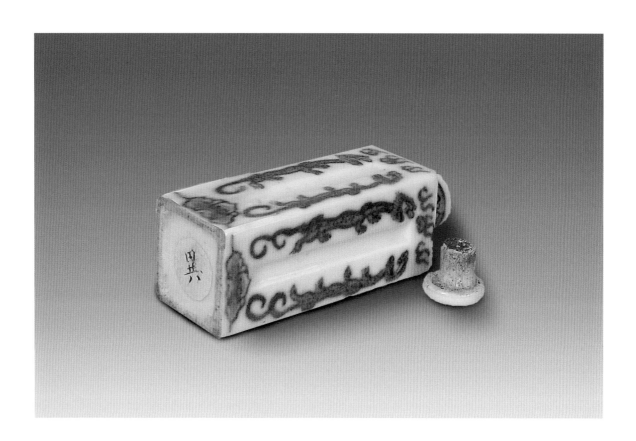

药瓶

近现代

瓷质

边长 2.6 厘米，通高 8.6 厘米

Medicine Bottle

Modern Times

Porcelain

Side Length 2.6 cm/ Height 8.6 cm

方瓶形，盛药器具。该藏品为我馆收藏的南翔张志方中药室红木药箱内配瓷药瓶之一，青花瓷，双龙戏珠纹，平底直口，上配瓷瓶盖，每个瓶盖上粘有药名标签，做工精细，造型美观，保存基本完好。1959年入藏。

中华医学会 / 上海中医药博物馆藏

The square bottle was for storing medicine. It is one of the porcelain medicine bottles equipped in the mahogany medicine chest in Zhang Zhifang Traditional Chinese Medicine Store at Nanxiang. The blue and white porcelain bottle is decorated with the design of two dragons playing a fireball. It has a flat bottom and a straight mouth and each porcelain cover is pasted a tag of medicine name. Its craft is exquisite and elegant. The bottle is still in good condition. It was collected in the year 1959.

Preserved in Chinese Medical Association/ Museum of Chinese Medicine, Shanghai University of Traditional Chinese Medicine

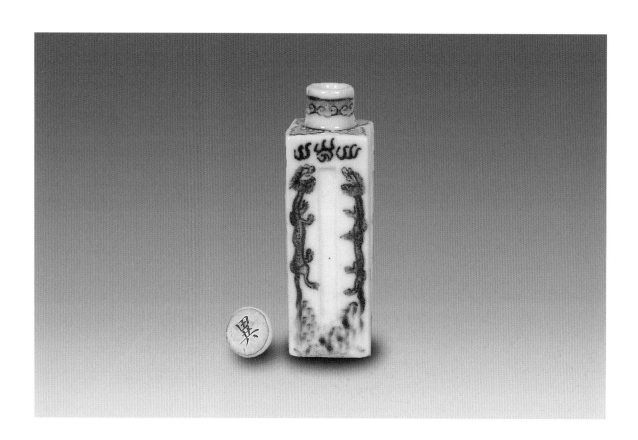

药瓶

近现代

瓷质

边长 2.6 厘米，通高 8.6 厘米

Medicine Bottle

Modern Times

Porcelain

Side Length 2.6 cm/ Height 8.6 cm

方瓶形，盛药器具。该藏品为我馆收藏的南翔张志方中药室红木药箱内配瓷药瓶之一，青花瓷，双龙戏珠纹，平底直口，上配瓷瓶盖，每个瓶盖上粘有药名标签，做工精细，造型美观，保存基本完好。1959年入藏。

中华医学会/上海中医药博物馆藏

The square bottle was for storing medicine. It is one of the porcelain medicine bottles equipped in the mahogany medicine chest in Zhang Zhifang Traditional Chinese Medicine Store at Nanxiang. The blue and white porcelain bottle is decorated with the design of two dragons playing a fireball. It has a flat bottom and a straight mouth and each porcelain cover is pasted a tag of medicine name. Its craft is exquisite and elegant. The bottle is still in good condition. It was collected in the year 1959.

Preserved in Chinese Medical Association/ Museum of Chinese Medicine, Shanghai University of Traditional Chinese Medicine

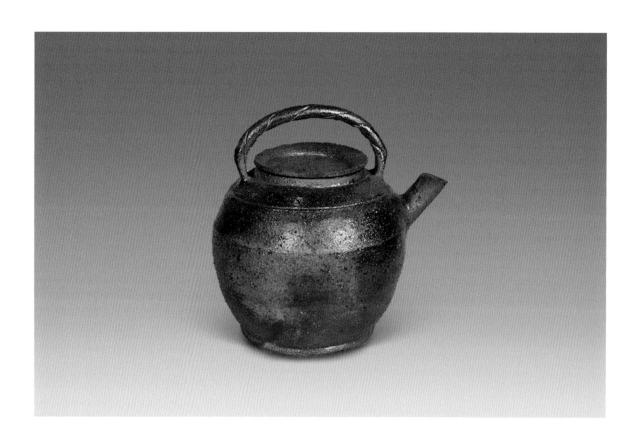

煎药壶

现代

陶质

口内径 7.1 厘米，口外径 9.2 厘米，腹径 13.5 厘米，通高 18 厘米

Kettle for Decocting Medicine

Modern Times

Pottery

Mouth Inner Diameter 7.1 cm/ Mouth Outer Diameter 9.2 cm/ Belly Diameter 13.5 cm/ Height 18 cm

壶形，为煎药器具。该藏品朱砂灰陶，表
面施亮釉，胎较薄，有提梁，肩部有壶嘴，
工艺粗糙，旋纹清晰，为现代广东民间煎
药用具。底部无款，有盖，保存基本完好。
1960 年入藏。

中华医学会 / 上海中医药博物馆藏

The kettle-shaped collection was for
dccocting crude herbal drugs. The cinnabar
grey pottery is covered with shining and
thin glaze. It has a hoop handle and a spout
on its shoulder. The craft is rough but it
is covered with distinct rotation patterns.
It was utilized for Guangdong folks to
decoct crude herbal drugs in modern times.
The kettle has a cover and there are no
inscriptions at the bottom. The bottle is still
in good condition. It was collected in the
year 1960.

Preserved in Chinese Medical Association/
Museum of Chinese Medicine, Shanghai
University of Traditional Chinese Medicine

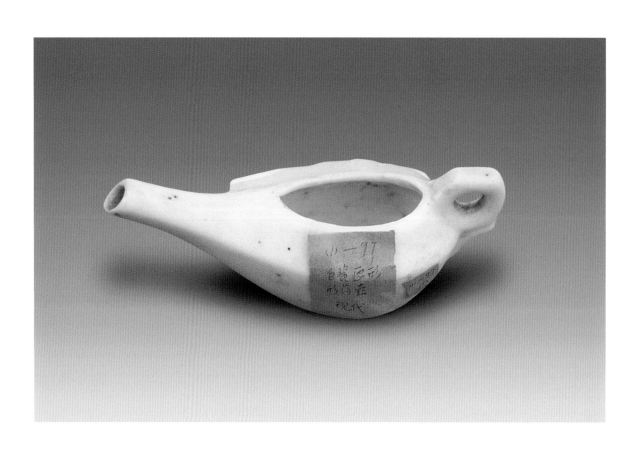

白瓷匜形药壶

近代

瓷质

长 12 厘米，通高 4.9 厘米，重 60 克

壶口：长 3 厘米，宽 2.2 厘米

壶底：长 4.5 厘米，底径宽 3 厘米

White Porcelain Medicine Pot in the Shape of Yi (Vessel)

Modern Times

Porcelain

Length 12 cm/ Height 4.9 cm/ Weight 60 g

Mouth of the Pot: Length3 cm/ Width 2.2 cm

Bottom of the Pot: Length 4.5 cm/ Width 3 cm

匜形，一些危重病人的中药煎剂常需要灌服。

广东中医药博物馆藏

The porcelain pot is in the shape of Yi (vessel). It was utilized for critical patients to take decocted medicine.

Preserved in Guangdong Chinese Medicine Museum

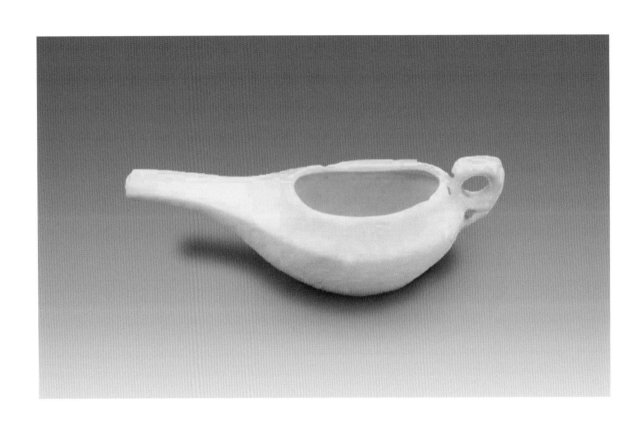

白瓷匜形药壶

近代

瓷质

长 16.2 厘米，通高 6.1 厘米，重 127 克

壶口：长 6.3 厘米，宽 3.1 厘米

壶底：长 6.3 厘米，宽 4.3 厘米

White Porcelain Medicine Pot in the Shape of Yi (Vessel)

Modern Times

Porcelain

Length 16.2 cm/ Height 6.1 cm/ Weight 127 g

Mouth of the Pot: Length 6.3 cm/ Width 3.1 cm

Bottom of the Pot: Length 6.3 cm/ Width 4.3 cm

匜形，一些危重病人的中药煎剂常需要灌服。

广东中医药博物馆藏

The porcelain pot is in the shape of Yi (vessel). It was utilized for critical patients to take decocted medicine.

Preserved in Guangdong Chinese Medicine Museum

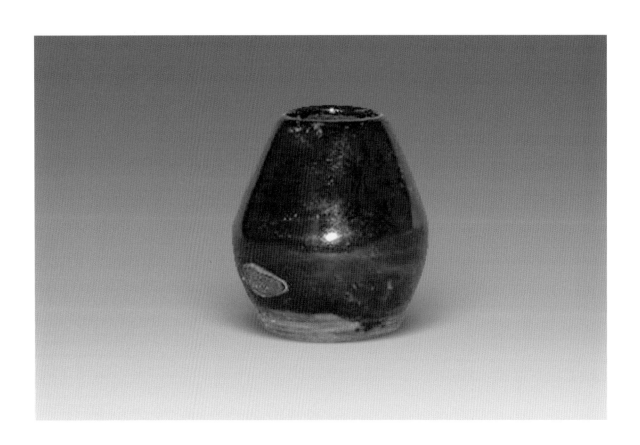

黑釉拔火罐

近代

瓷质

口径 3.6 厘米，底径 5 厘米，高 7.8 厘米，重 150 克

Black Glazed Cupping Pot

Modern Times

Porcelain

Mouth Diameter 3.6 cm/ Bottom Diameter 5 cm/ Height 7.8 cm/ Weight 150 g

弇口，鼓腹，圈足，腹下部有一棱形印记，通体黑釉，
圈足无釉。医疗器具。保存完整，2001 年 9 月入藏。
陕西省西安市古玩市场征集。

陕西医史博物馆藏

The pot has a small contracted mouth, a ring
foot and a bulging belly whose lower part has
a prismatic mark. It is wholly covered with
black glaze except the foot and was utilized as a
medical utensil. The pot, which is still kept intact,
was collected from the antique market in Xi'an,
Shaanxi Province in September, 2001.

Preserved in Shaanxi Museum of Medical History

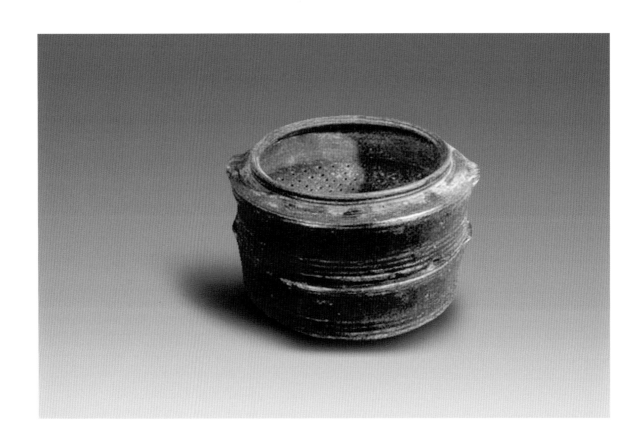

陶质蒸笼

近代

陶质

直径 32 厘米，高 18 厘米

Ceramic Food Steamer

Modern Times

Pottery

Diameter 32 cm/ Height 18 cm

字母口，无盖，折肩，扁圆柱形，平底，底上有排列规则的透气孔，圆圈足。用于蒸制食物的器具。

西藏博物馆藏

The coverless flat column ware has two matching mouths, a folding shoulder, a flat bottom and a ring foot. The bottom is provided with ventilating holes arranged in a regular pattern. The ware was utilized for steaming food.

Preserved in Tibet Museum

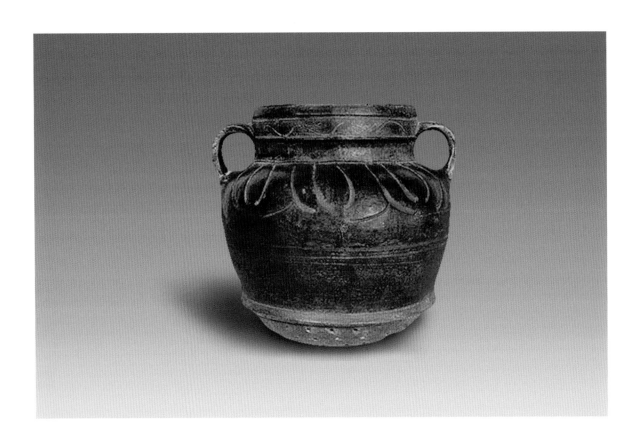

陶质双耳蒸器

近代

陶质

最大直径 21 厘米，高 21 厘米

Ceramic Food Steamer with Two Handles

Modern Times

Pottery

The Maximum Diameter 21 cm/ Height 21 cm

敛口，平沿，短颈，溜肩，鼓腹渐收至底，平底，

圈足，颈肩部刻有花纹，左右相对有耳一对。

用于蒸制食物的器具。

西藏博物馆藏

The utensil has a contracted mouth, a flat edge, a short neck, a smooth shoulder, a bulging belly, a flat bottom and a ring foot. The neck and shoulder are carved with flower patterns and there is a handle on each side. The utensil was utilized for steaming food.

Preserved in Tibet Museum

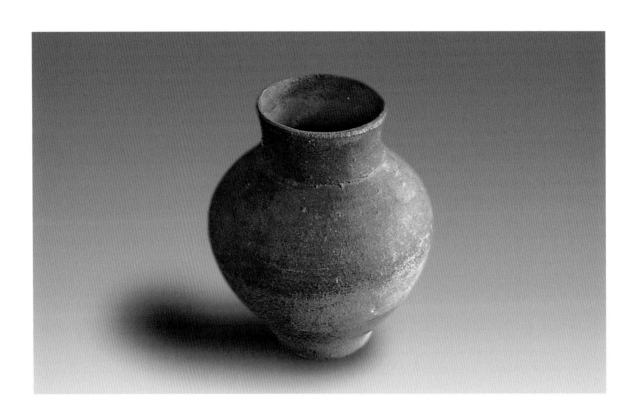

罐

近代

陶质

口径 6 厘米，高 12 厘米

Pot

Modern Times

Pottery

Mouth Diameter 6 cm/ Height 12 cm

口稍敞，直颈，鼓腹，平底，上半部施黄釉。由民间征集。

成都中医药大学中医药传统文化博物馆藏

The pot has a slightly flared mouth, a straight neck, a bulging belly and a flat bottom. The upper half of the pot is covered with yellow glaze, It was collected from a private owner. Preserved in Museum of Traditional Chinese Medicine Culture, Chengdu University of Traditional Chinese Medicine

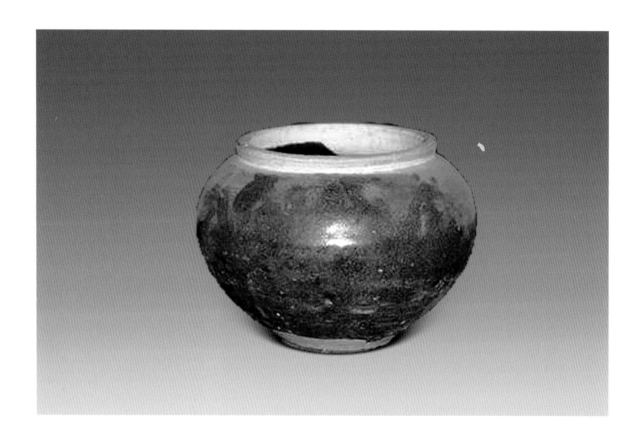

棕釉罐

近代

瓷质

口径 9.5 厘米，底径 5.4 厘米，通高 9.4 厘米，重 500 克

Brown Glazed Pot

Modern Times

Porcelain

Mouth Diameter 9.5 cm/ Bottom Diameter 5.4 cm/ Height 9.4 cm/ Weight 500 g

直口，圆肩，圆腹，圈足，口底无釉。生活器具。
陕西省澄城县征集。

陕西医史博物馆藏

The pot has a straight mouth, a round shoulder, a belly and a ring foot. The mouth is unglazed. The pot, which was utilized as a life utensil. was collected from Chengcheng County, Shaanxi Province.

Preserved in Shaanxi Museum of Medical History

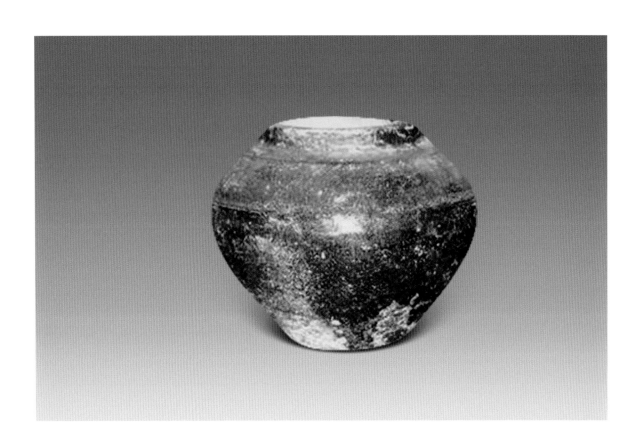

黑釉瓷罐

近代

瓷质

口径 8.5 厘米，底径 7.5 厘米，通高 11 厘米，重 600 克

Black Glazed Porcelain Pot

Modern Times

Porcelain

Mouth Diameter 8.5 cm/ Bottom Diameter 7.5 cm/ Height 11 cm/ Weight 600 g

直口，鼓腹，平底，肩腹之间有二圈细棱。盛贮器，口稍残。

陕西医史博物馆藏

The pot has a straight mouth, a bulging belly and a flat bottom. There are two circles of thin ridges between its shoulder and belly. Its mouth is slightly damaged. The pot was utilized for storing.

Preserved in Shaanxi Museum of Medical History

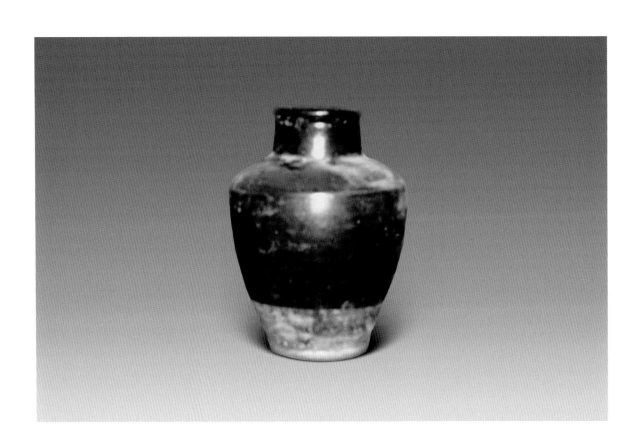

黑瓷罐

近代

瓷质

口径 8 厘米，底径 9 厘米，通高 22 厘米，重 1300 克

Black Porcelain Pot

Modern Times

Porcelain

Mouth Diameter 8 cm/ Bottom Diameter 9 cm/ Height 22 cm/ Weight 1300 g

圆口，直颈，斜腹，斜肩，圈足，下腹无釉黑粗瓷。盛贮器，完整无损。

陕西医史博物馆藏

The pot, which is roughly covered with black glaze except its lower belly, has a round mouth, a straight neck, a sloping belly, a sloping shoulder and a ring foot. The pot was utilized for storing. It is still in good condition.

Preserved in Shaanxi Museum of Medical History

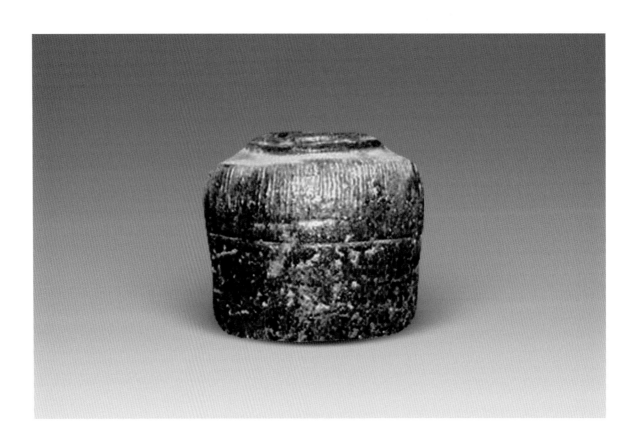

黑瓷罐

近代

瓷质

口径 11.5 厘米，底径 18 厘米，通高 18 厘米，重 1900 克

Black Porcelain Pot

Modern Times

Porcelain

Mouth Diameter 11.5 cm/ Bottom Diameter 18 cm/ Height 18 cm/ Weight 1900 g

子母口，平肩直腹，平底，肩、腹之间有一圈竖道。
盛贮器，完整无损。

陕西医史博物馆藏

The pot has a square shoulder, a flat bottom, a straight belly and two matching mouths. A carved round pattern as a vertical strip is between the shoulder and the belly. The pot was utilized for storing. It is still in good condition.

Preserved in Shaanxi Museum of Medical History

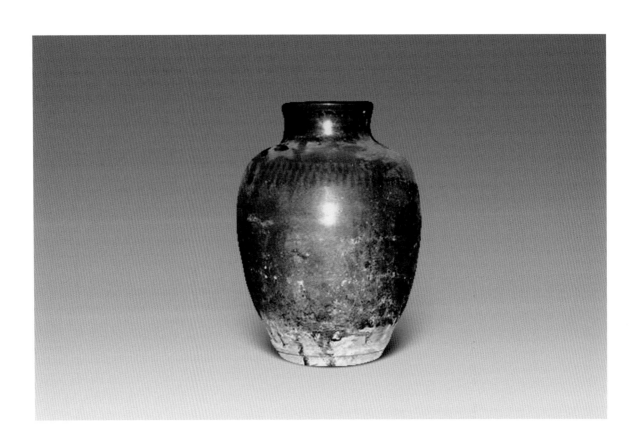

黑瓷罐

近代

瓷质

口径 10 厘米，底径 26 厘米，通高 11 厘米，重 2050 克

Black Porcelain Pot

Modern Times

Porcelain

Mouth Diameter 10 cm/ Bottom Diameter 26 cm/ Height 11 cm/ Weight 2050 g

小喇叭口，直径，小圆腹，下腹有一圈凸棱，平底。

盛贮器，完整无损。

陕西医史博物馆藏

The pot has a small flared mouth, a flat bottom and a small round belly under which is a circle of raised ridges. The pot was utilized for storing. It is still in good condition.

Preserved in Shaanxi Museum of Medical History

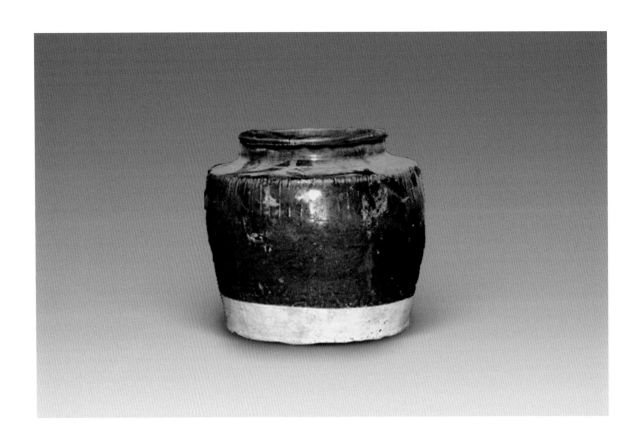

黑瓷罐

近代

瓷质

口径 13.5 厘米，底径 18 厘米，通高 7 厘米，重 1550 克

Black Porcelain Pot

Modern Times

Porcelain

Mouth Diameter 13.5 cm/ Bottom Diameter 18 cm/ Height 7 cm/ Weight 1550 g

圆唇，平肩，直腹，平底，下腹一寸高处白胎无釉。盛贮器，完整无损。

陕西医史博物馆藏

The pot has a round mouth, a flat shoulder, a flat bottom and a straight belly. The part, which is 3.33 cm high above the bottom, is white body and unglazed. The pot was utilized for storing. It is still in good condition.

Preserved in Shaanxi Museum of Medical History

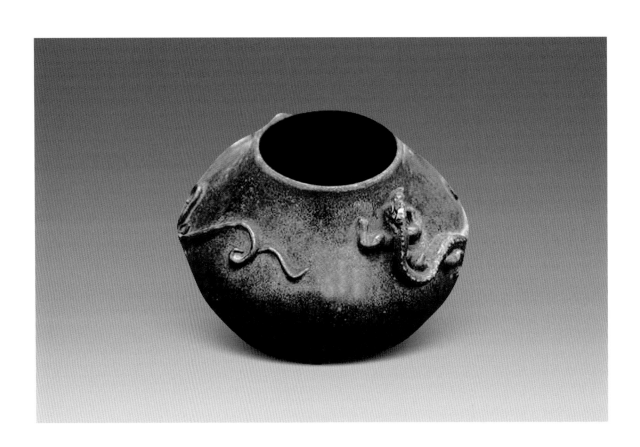

堆花双龙纹瓷罐

近代

瓷质

口外径 12.3 厘米，底径 13.28 厘米，腹径 25.7 厘米，腹深 15.9 厘米，重 3500 克

Porcelain Pot with Paste-on-paste Design of Two Dragons

Modern Times

Porcelain

Mouth Outer Diameter 12.3 cm/ Bottom Diameter 13.28 cm/ Belly Diameter 25.7 cm/ Belly Depth 13.9 cm/ Weight 3500 g

瓷质容器，生活器具。

广东中医药博物馆藏

The porcelain vessel was utilized as a life utensil.

Preserved in Guangdong Chinese Medicine Museum

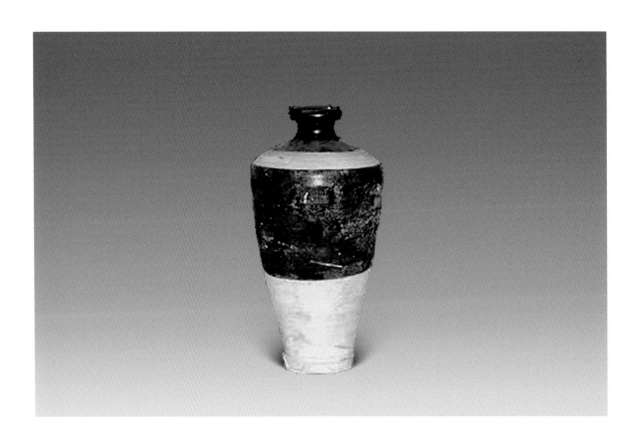

黑瓷瓶

近代

瓷质

口径 4 厘米，底径 5 厘米，通高 19 厘米，重 450 克

Black Porcelain Vase

Modern Times

Porcelain

Mouth Diameter 4 cm/ Bottom Diameter 5 cm/ Height 19 cm/ Weight 450 g

圆唇，斜肩，斜腹，圈足，肩有 1.5 厘米白胎，
下腹无釉。盛贮器，口残。

陕西医史博物馆藏

The pot has a slightly damaged round mouth, a
sloping shoulder, a sloping belly and a ring foot. A
part of 1.5 cm wide of the shoulder is white body.
The lower part belly is unglazed. The pot was
utilized for storing.

Preserved in Shaanxi Museum of Medical History

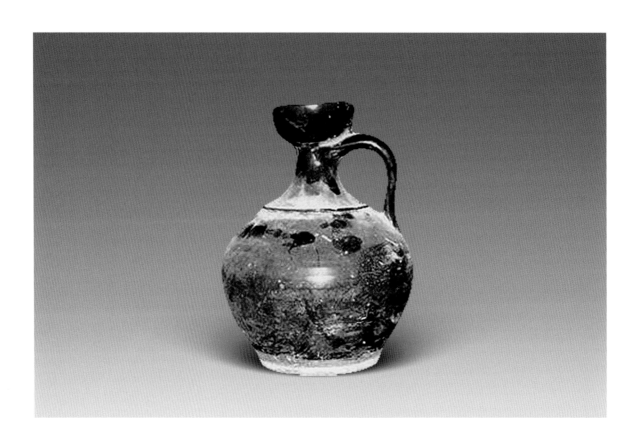

黑釉执壶

近代

瓷质

口径 7.2 厘米，底径 10.2 厘米，通高 20 厘米，重 1150 克

Black Glazed Pot

Modern Times

Porcelain

Mouth Diameter 7.2 cm/ Bottom Diameter 10.2 cm/ Height 20 cm/ Weight 1150 g

深盘口，短颈，肩有一凸棱，一执，圆腹，圈足，足底无釉。生活器具。保存完整，陕西省澄城县征集。

陕西医史博物馆藏

The pot has a deep mouth, a short neck, a round belly and an unglazed ring foot. There is an arris and one handle on the shoulder. The pot, which was utilized as a life utensil. It was collected from Chengcheng County, Shaanxi Province. It is still in good condition.

Preserved in Shaanxi Museum of Medical History

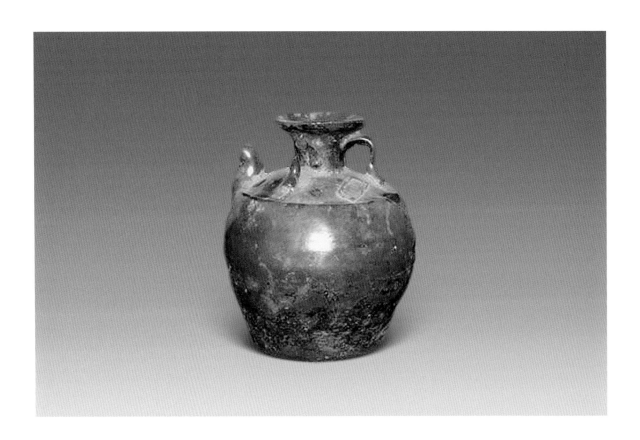

酱釉瓷壶

近代

瓷质

口径 5.9 厘米，底径 7.2 厘米，通高 12.8 厘米，重 400 克

Brown Glazed Porcelain Pot

Modern Times

Porcelain

Mouth Diameter 5.9 cm/ Bottom Diameter 7.2 cm/ Height 12.8 cm/ Weight 400 g

小喇叭口，短颈，平肩，圆腹，浅圈足，肩部有三耳，
并有一流，流口残，腹有裂痕。酱釉。生活器具，
1999 年 12 月 8 日入藏，陕西省澄城县征集。

陕西医史博物馆藏

The pot, covered with brown glaze, has a small
flared mouth, a short neck, a flat shoulder, a
shallow ring foot and a round belly with cracks.
There are three handles and one damaged spout
on its shoulder. The pot, which was utilized as
a life utensil. was collected from Chengcheng
County, Shaanxi Province on December 8th,
1999.

Preserved in Shaanxi Museum of Medical History

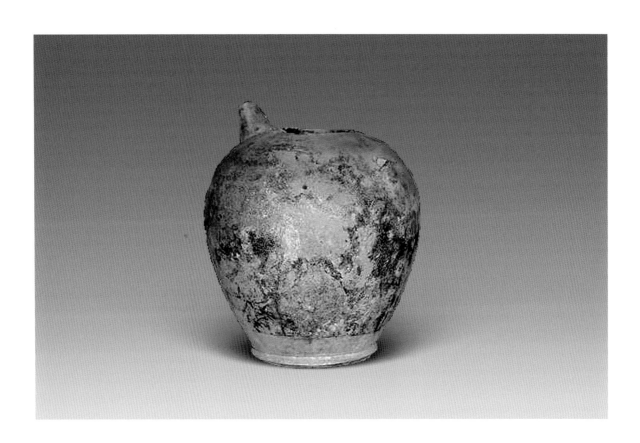

瓷壶

近代

瓷质

口径 6.5 厘米，底径 10 厘米，通高 17 厘米，重 1510 克

Porcelain Pot

Modern Times

Pottery

Mouth Diameter 6.5 cm/ Bottom Diameter 10 cm/ Height 17 cm/ Weight 1510 g

圆肩，圆腹，平底，肩上有一壶流。口把残。生活用器。

陕西医史博物馆藏

The pot has a round shoulder, a round belly and a flat bottom. There is a damaged spout on its shoulder. It was utilized as a life utensil.

Preserved in Shaanxi Museum of Medical History

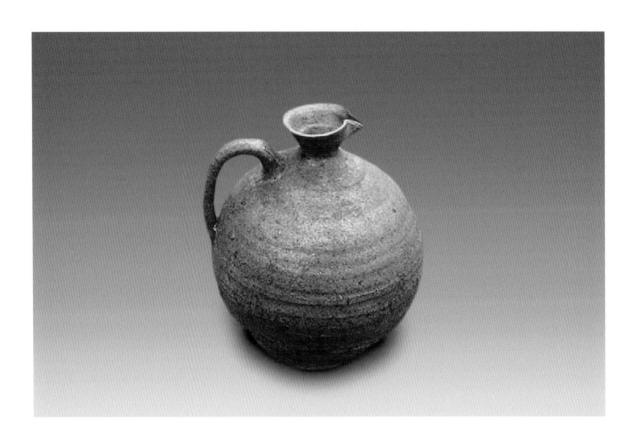

黄釉陶壶

近代

陶质

口外径 7.37 厘米，腹径 20.5 厘米，底径 14.78 厘米，通高 25.4 厘米，重 2500 克

Yellow Glazed Pottery Pot

Modern Times

Pottery

Mouth Outer Diameter 7.37 cm/ Belly Diameter 20.5 cm/ Bottom Diameter 14.78 cm/ Height 25.4 cm/ Weight 2500 g

大腹，小口，无盖，带把。生活用品。

广东中医药博物馆藏

The pottery pot has a big belly a small mouth, and a lidless handle. It was utilized as a life utensil.

Preserved in Guangdong Chinese Medicine Museum

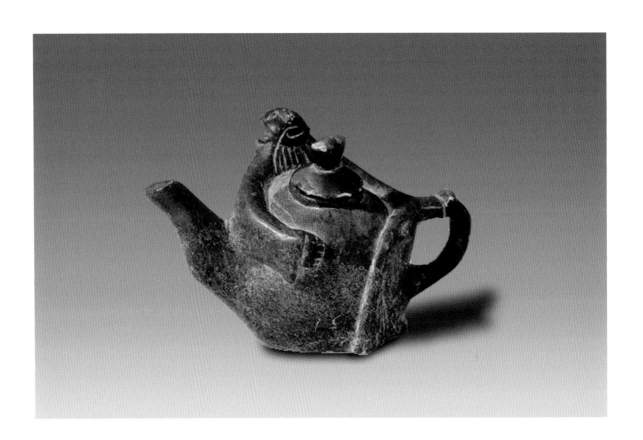

长寿酒壶

近代

瓷质

直径 13 厘米，高 8.3 厘米

Longevity Wine Pot

Modern Times

Porcelain

Diameter 13 cm/ Height 8.3 cm

鼓腹，一个长须老翁仰天长啸，双臂环抱壶腹，有盖，盖上有纽，直流，把与流相对，平底。

西藏博物馆藏

The pot has a bulging belly. A long-bearded old man painted on the pot was yelling to the sky with his arms held around the pot belly. The pot has a lid with a handle on it. The pot bottom is flat.

Preserved in Tibet Museum

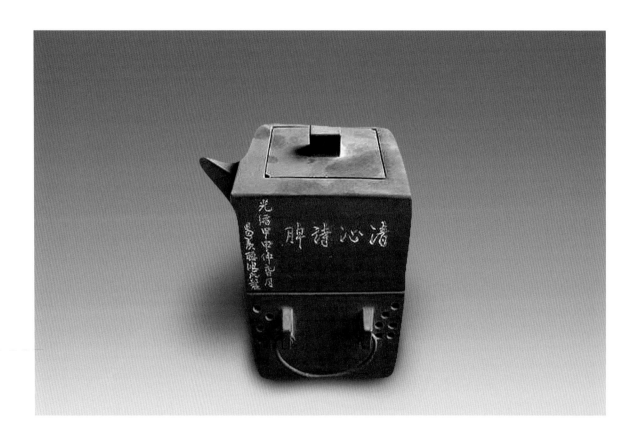

茶壶

晚清

紫砂

口径 5.8 厘米，宽 7 厘米，高 15 厘米

Teapot

Late Qing Dynasty

Red Porcelain

Mouth Diameter 5.8 cm/ Width 7 cm/ Height 15 cm

有"清心诗脾"等字样。晚清名医余听鸿

（1847—1907）监制方形雕空紫砂茶壶。

江苏省中医药博物馆藏

The teapot is incised with the Chinese characters "Qing Xin Shi Pi". The making of the square red porcelain teapot in piercing carving was supervised by the famous doctor Yu Tinghong (1847-1907) in the Late Qing Dynasty.

Preserved in Jiangsu Museum of Traditional Chinese Medicine

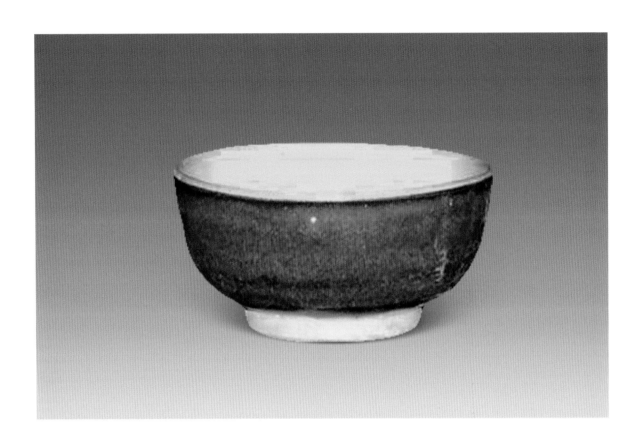

粗瓷小碗

近代

瓷质

口径 8.5 厘米，底径 4.5 厘米，通高 3.8 厘米，重 150 克

Small Stoneware Bowl

Modern Times

Porcelain

Mouth Diameter 8.5 cm/ Bottom Diameter 4.5 cm/ Height 3.8 cm/ Weight 150 g

碗内为白釉，外为黑釉，平底圈足。食器，完整无损。

陕西医史博物馆藏

The inner surface of the bowl is covered with opal glaze and the outer part is black glaze. It has a flat bottom and a ring foot and was utilized as tableware. The bowl is still in good condition.

Preserved in Shaanxi Museum of Medical History

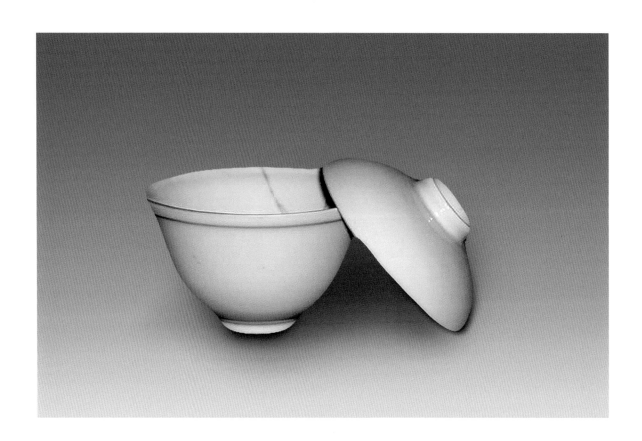

白瓷盖碗杯

近代

瓷质

口径 11 厘米，底径 3.8 厘米，通高 9.4 厘米，重 200 克

碗：高 6.3 厘米

White Porcelain Tureen Cup

Modern Times

Porcelain

Mouth Diameter 11 cm/ Bottom Diameter 3.8 cm/ Height 9.4 cm/ Weight 200 g

Cup: Height 6.3 cm

敞口，直斜腹，圈足，带一盖，盖足内和圈足内
有一青花印，通体白釉，碗部沿呈黄色。碗有裂痕。
生活器具。陕西省咸阳市文物市场征集。

陕西医史博物馆藏

The bowl has a flared mouth, a straight sloping
belly, a ring foot and a cap. A blue and white
imprint is at the inner foot of the bowl and cap
respectively. It is wholly covered with white glaze
and its rim is light yellow. There are some cracks
on its surface. The bowl, which was utilized as a
life utensil, was collected from the cultural relics
market in Xianyang City, Shaanxi Province.
Preserved in Shaanxi Museum of Medical History

美人枕

清末民初

瓷质

长 33 厘米，宽 13 厘米，高 21 厘米

胎质灰白，施化妆土和蓝色、黄褐色透明釉。女人为侧卧状、头部上扬，上衣为蓝色，裤子为黄褐色带
墨点花圈，缠足。磁县出土。

磁州窑博物馆藏

Beauty-shaped Pillow

Late Qing Dynasty or Early Republican Period

Porcelain

Length 33 cm/ Width 13 cm/ Height 21 cm

The pillow surface is grey and white, and is covered with engobe and blue and tawny transparent glaze.
The foot-binding lady, wearing a blue coat and tawny trousers decorated with wreaths enclosed by white
spots, is lying on her side and raising her head upward. The pillow was collected from Cixian County.
Preserved in Cizhou Kiln Museum

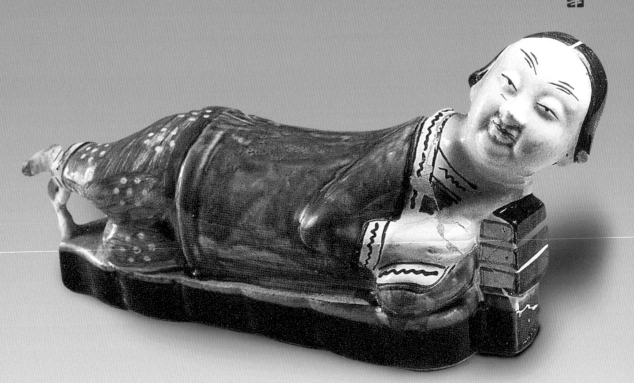

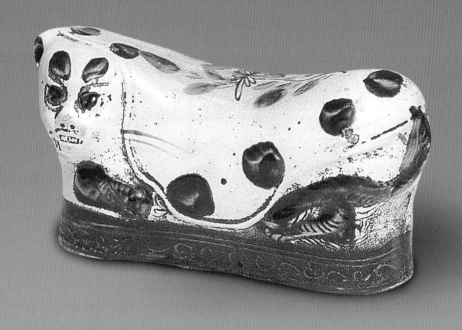

虎形枕

近代

瓷质

长 26 厘米，宽 10 厘米，高 12 厘米

为近代北方民窑瓷器，虎枕右耳有一圆孔，可将
冷水注入枕内，有降温作用。

北京中医药大学中医药博物馆藏

Modern Times

Porcelain

Length 26 cm/ Width 10 cm/ Height 12 cm

The porcelain pillow is of the north folk kilns in
modern times. There is a round hole on the right
ear of the tiger where cold water can be injected
for cooling purpose.

Preserved in the Museum of Chinese Medicine,
Beijing University of Chinese Medicine

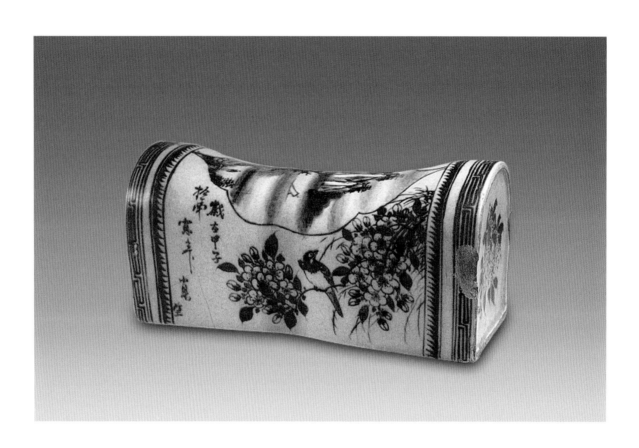

上圆下方青花枕

清末民初

瓷质

长 36 厘米，宽 14 厘米，高 14 厘米

Blue-and-white Glazed Pillow with Round Top and Square Bottom

Late Qing Dynasty or Early Republican Period

Porcelain

Length 36 cm/ Width 14 cm/ Height 14 cm

胎质灰白坚硬，施化妆土、透明釉，通体为灰白色，底部釉色
与枕面相同，有一个小气孔。枕面全为青花，共有五个装饰部
位：枕面两端绘回纹，中间有空白相间；枕顶部画水山人物；
一侧面绘菊花小鸟，有墨书"菊有秋香"四字，署款为："岁在
甲子于南窗之下，小泉涂"；另一侧绘花卉一枝，枝上落一小鸟，
墨书"岁在甲子于南窗之下，小泉涂"；两端面各绘佛手一个。
磁县城内滏阳街出土。

私人藏

The hard surface of the pillow is grey and white, and is covered
with engobe and transparent glaze. The entire pillow is off-
white. The glazing color of the bottom is identical to that of the
pillow surface. The pillow has a spilehole. The pillow surface
is completely decorated with blue and white patterns. There are
five parts of the patterns in total: both ends are painted with hui
patterns alternating with the white strip; the top is decorated
with the design of landscape and figures; the obverse side is the
picture of chrysanthemum and birds, with four Chinese characters
"Ju You Qiu Xiang" and the inscriptions "Sui Zai Jia Zi Yu Nan
Chuang Zhi Xia, Xiao Quan Tu " ; the other side is painted with
a branch of flowers and plants, with a bird on it; the left and the
right ends are respectively painted with one fingered citron. The
pillow was collected from Fuyang Avenue, Cixian County.
Preserved by a Private Owner

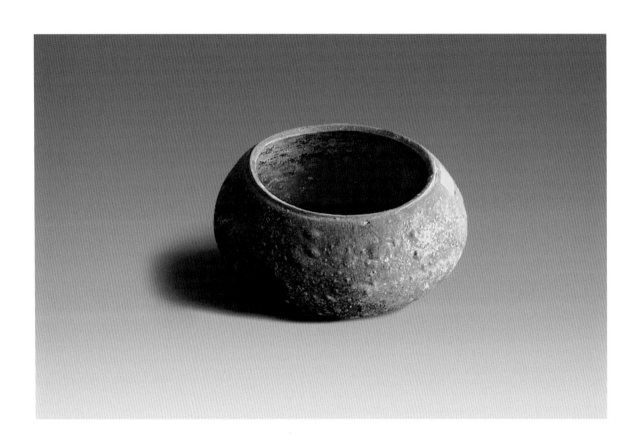

洗

现代

瓷质

口径 18 厘米，高 10 厘米

Washbowl

Modern Times

Porcelain

Mouth Diameter 18 cm/ Height 10 cm

侈口，彭腹，底微圆，施黄釉，略有脱落。由成都市考古队调拨。

成都中医药大学中医药传统文化博物馆藏

The wash bowl has a wide flared mouth, a bulgy belly and a round bottom. The surface is covered with yellow glaze and some of the yellow glaze slightly Peels off. It was allocated from Chengdu Archaeological Team.

Preserved in Museum of Traditional Chinese Medicine Culture, Chengdu University of Traditional Chinese Medicine

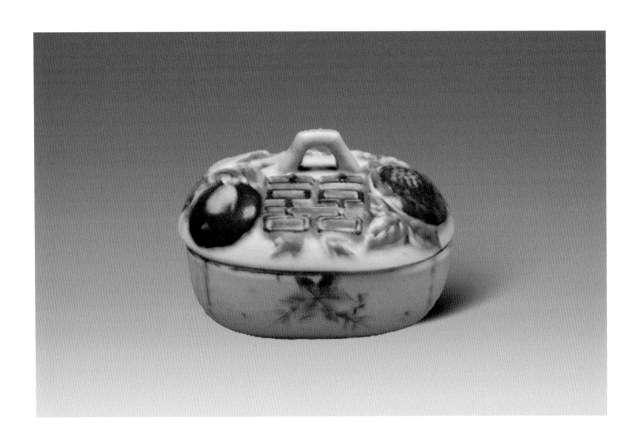

皂盒

民国时期

瓷质

长 11.8 厘米，宽 8.8 厘米，高 9.4 厘米

Soapbox

Republican Period

Porcelain

Length 11.8 cm/ Width 8.8 cm/ Height 9.4 cm

器形完整，长方形，四角为弧形，饰彩花纹，盖上堆塑五彩水果纹及民间常有的"囍"字纹，颜色鲜艳，色彩丰富，桥形纽，盖与器身有子母口相合，用于盛放皂胰，是日常生活中使用的卫生用具。1998 年四川省文物总店调拨。

成都中医药大学中医药传统文化博物馆藏

The soap box is rectangular and intact. The four corners are arch-shaped. Its surface is decorated with colorful flowers. The lid is paste-on-paste decoration of multicolored fruits and is painted with the usual folk pattern of the Chinese character "Xi", meaning Double happiness. The whole design is rich and bright in color. The knob of the box is shaped like a bridge. The two matching mouths connect the lid and the box tightly. This sanitary appliance was used in daily life for storing soap. It was allocated from Sichuan Provincial Cultural Relics Store in 1998.

Preserved in Museum of Traditional Chinese Medicine Culture, Chengdu University of Traditional Chinese Medicine

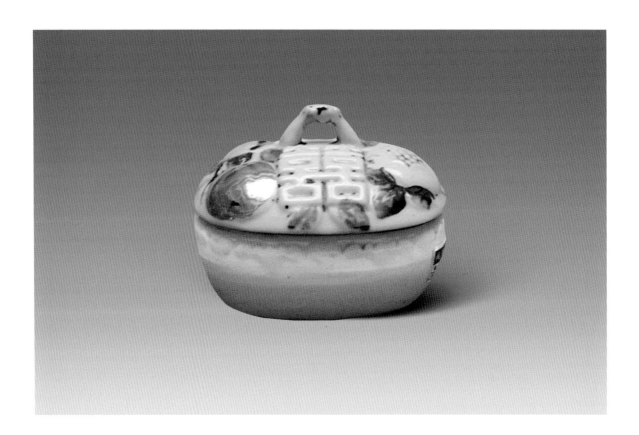

皂盒

民国时期

瓷质

长 11.8 厘米，宽 8.8 厘米，高 9.4 厘米

Soapbox

Republican Period

Porcelain

Length 11.8 cm/ Width 8.8 cm/ Height 9.4 cm

长方形，四角为弧形，饰彩花纹，盖上堆塑
五彩水果纹及"囍"字纹。四川省文物总店
调拨。

成都中医药大学中医药传统文化博物馆藏

The soapbox is rectangular and its four
corners are arch-shaped. Its surface is
decorated with colorful flowers. The lid is
paste-on-paste decoration of multicolored
fruits with the usual pattern of the Chinese
character "Xi", meaning double happiness.
It was allocated from Sichuan Provincial
Cultural Relics Store.
Preserved in Museum of Traditional Chinese
Medicine Culture, Chengdu University of
Traditional Chinese Medicine

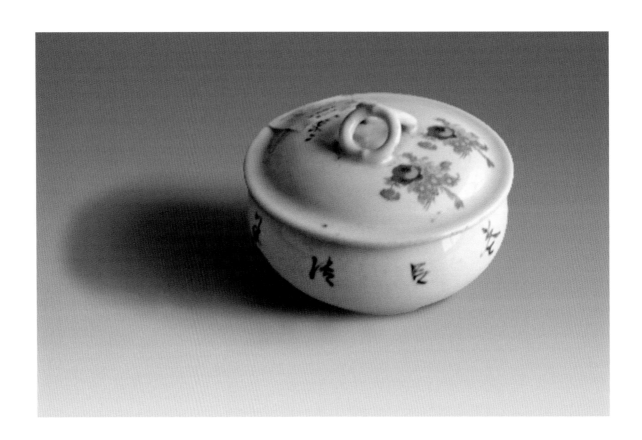

皂盒

民国时期

瓷质

直径 9.5 厘米，高 7 厘米

Soapbox

Republican Period

Porcelain

Diameter 9.5 cm/ Height 7 cm

圆形，敛口，鼓腹，平底，圈足，腹上饰五彩花卉纹，墨书"益气清香"几个字，盖较平，上有彩色花卉纹和"八大山人"几个墨字，由两个小圆环相搭成纽，十分别致。盛放皂胰的用具。由四川省文物总店征集。

成都中医药大学中医药传统文化博物馆藏

The round box has a contracting mouth, a bulgy belly, a flat bottom and a ring foot. The belly of the box is decorated with the patterns of flowers and plants and painted with some Chinese characters "Yi Qi Qing Xiang". The lid is a little bit flat and decorated with the patterns of colorful flowers and plants plus some Chinese characters "Ba Da Shan Ren" in ink. The knob, made of two joined little rings, is very unique and exquisite. This item which was utilized for storing soap, was collected from Sichuan Provincial Cultural Relics Store.

Preserved in Museum of Traditional Chinese Medicine Culture, Chengdu University of Traditional Chinese Medicine

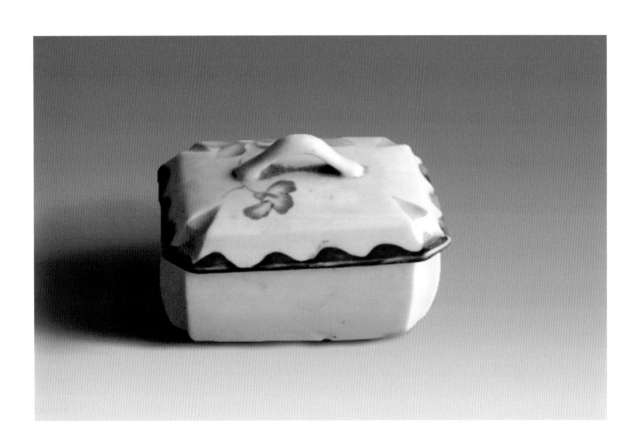

皂盒

民国时期

瓷质

长 10 厘米，宽 9 厘米，高 5.5 厘米

Soapbox

Republican Period

Porcelain

Length 10 cm/ Width 9 cm/ Height 5.5 cm

长方形，四角切边，盖沿为荷瓣形，板桥纽。由民间征集。

　　成都中医药大学中医药传统文化博物馆藏

The soapbox is rectangular and its four corners are edge trimming. The edge of the lid is in the shape of a lotus petal. The knob is shaped as a slab bridge. The box was collected from a private owner.

Preserved in Museum of Traditional Chinese Medicine Culture, Chengdu University of Traditional Chinese Medicine

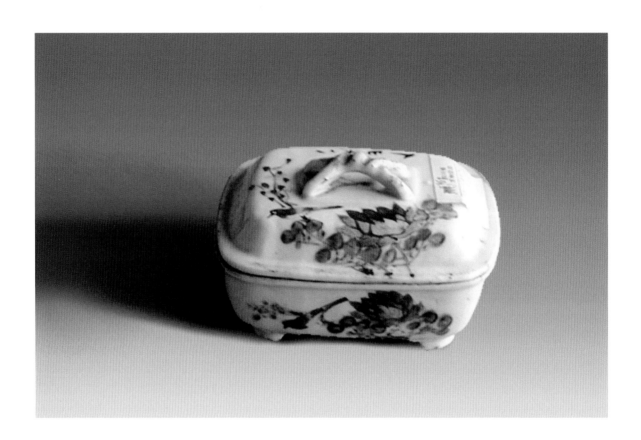

皂盒

民国时期

瓷质

长 11 厘米，宽 8.5 厘米，高 7.5 厘米

Soapbox

Republican Period

Porcelain

Length 11 cm/ Width 8.5 cm/ Height 7.5 cm

器身呈方鼎形，平口直腹，平底，四个弧形足，饰彩色花鸟纹饰及"八大山人"等墨字，盖上有枝叶形纽。由四川省文物总店征集。

成都中医药大学中医药传统文化博物馆藏

The soapbox is in the shape of a square Ding, has a plain top, a straight belly, a flat bottom and four arch-shaped feet. The surface is decorated with the patterns of colorful flowers and birds and some Chinese characters "Ba Da Shan Ren" written in ink. The lid has a leaf-shaped knob. The box was collected from Sichuan Provincial Cultural Relics Store.

Preserved in Museum of Traditional Chinese Medicine Culture, Chengdu University of Traditional Chinese Medicine

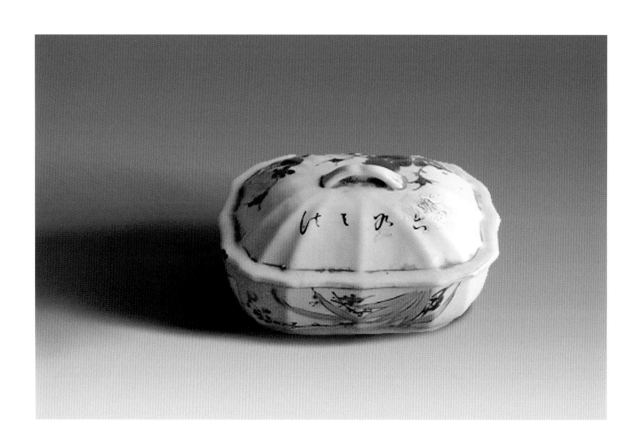

皂盒

民国时期

瓷质

长 11.5 厘米，宽 9 厘米，高 6.5 厘米

Soapbox

Republican Period

Porcelain

Length 11.5 cm/ Width 9 cm/ Height 6.5 cm

荷叶形，器盖与器身呈荷瓣形。器身为直口平底圈足，足底赤书有"江西黄礼和造"铭，底内有五个圆锥形的凸起，便于固定皂胰，外壁饰彩色花卉纹，盖上饰有花卉纹，板桥形纽。由四川省文物总店征集。

成都中医药大学中医药传统文化博物馆藏

The soapbox is in the shape of a lotus-petal. The box has a straight mouth, a flat bottom and a ring foot on which inscriptions "Made by Huang Lihe in Jiangxi Province" are red painted. There are five conoid protruding points at the bottom to keep the soap inside the box. The exterior surface is decorated with the patterns of colorful flowers and plants and the lid is decorated with flower designs. The knob is shaped like a bridge. The box was collected from Sichuan Provincial Cultural Relics Store.

Preserved in Museum of Traditional Chinese Medicine Culture, Chengdu University of Traditional Chinese Medicine

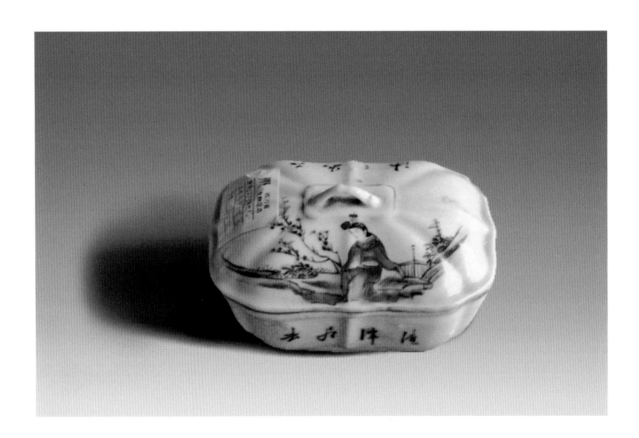

皂盒

民国时期

瓷质

长 11.5 厘米，宽 8.5 厘米，高 6 厘米

Soapbox

Republican Period

Porcelain

Length 11.5 cm/ Width 8.5 cm/ Height 6 cm

荷叶纹，器盖与器身呈荷瓣形，器身平口，腹微敛，圈足，足底有赤书"江西陈华珍出品"铭，内底有六个圆锥状凸起，用于固定皂胰，器身饰彩色人物和花卉纹，盖上亦饰彩色人物与花卉，板桥形纽，盖微残。由四川省文物总店征集。

成都中医药大学中医药传统文化博物馆藏

The soapbox is in the shape of a lotus-petal, The box has a plain top, a slightly contracting belly and a ring foot on which inscriptions "Made by Chen Huazhen in Jiangxi Province" are red painted. There are six conoid protruding points at the bottom to keep the soap inside the box. The exterior surface is decorated with the designs of colorful figures and the patterns of colorful flowers and plants and the lid is also decorated with the same designs and patterns. The knob is shaped like a bridge. The lid is slightly damaged. The box was collected from Sichuan Provincial Cultural Relics Store.

Preserved in Museum of Traditional Chinese Medicine Culture, Chengdu University of Traditional Chinese Medicine

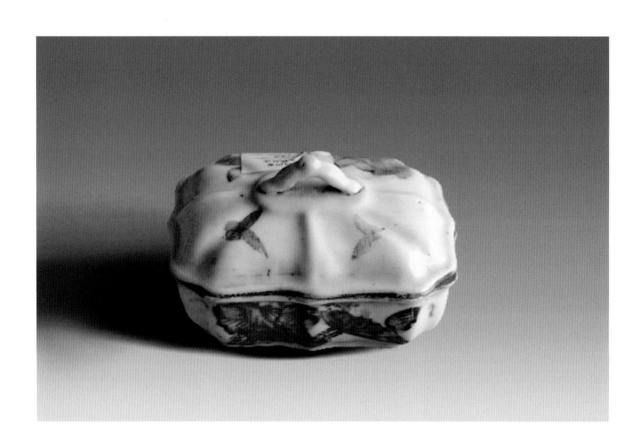

皂盒

民国时期

瓷质

长 10.5 厘米，宽 8 厘米，高 7 厘米

Soapbox

Republican Period

Porcelain

Length 10.5 cm/ Width 8 cm/ Height 7 cm

荷叶形，盖与器身呈荷瓣纹，饰有彩色花卉纹，花卉经脉由金色勾勒，桥形纽，器内底有六个圆锥状突起。由四川省文物总店征集。

成都中医药大学中医药传统文化博物馆藏

The box, in the shape of a lotus-petal, is decorated with the patterns of colorful flowers and plants whose veins are painted with golden color. It has a bridge-shaped knob. There are six conoid protruding parts at the bottom. It was collected from Sichuan Provincial Cultural Relics Store.

Preserved in Museum of Traditional Chinese Medicine Culture, Chengdu University of Traditional Chinese Medicine

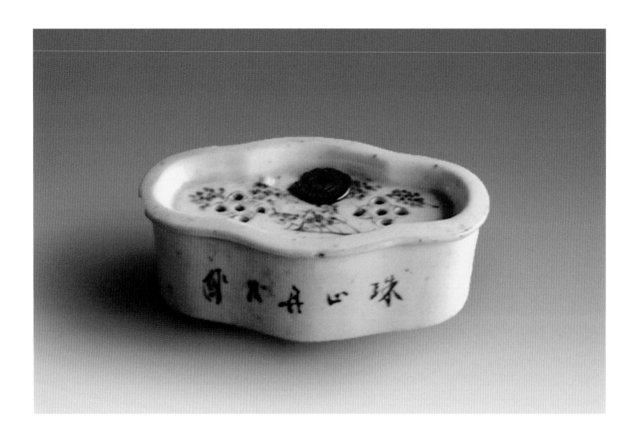

皂盒

民国时期

瓷质

长 11.5 厘米，宽 6.5 厘米，高 4 厘米

Soapbox

Republican Period

Porcelain

Length 11.5 cm/ Width 6.5 cm/ Height 4 cm

花瓣纹，直口平底圈足，饰彩色花卉纹，盖
内凹与器身相扣，上饰彩色花卉纹和两个圆
形的镂空万字孔。由四川省文物总店征集。

成都中医药大学中医药传统文化博物馆藏

The soapbox is in the shape of a petal, has a
straight mouth, a flat bottom and a ring foot and
is decorated with patterns of colorful flowers
and plants. The lid concaves downward and
buckles the body tightly. The whole box is
decorated with colorful flowers and plants
and two round engraving holes of swastika
designs. This item was collected from
Sichuan Provincial Cultural Relics Store.

Preserved in Museum of Traditional Chinese
Medicine Culture, Chengdu University of
Traditional Chinese Medicine

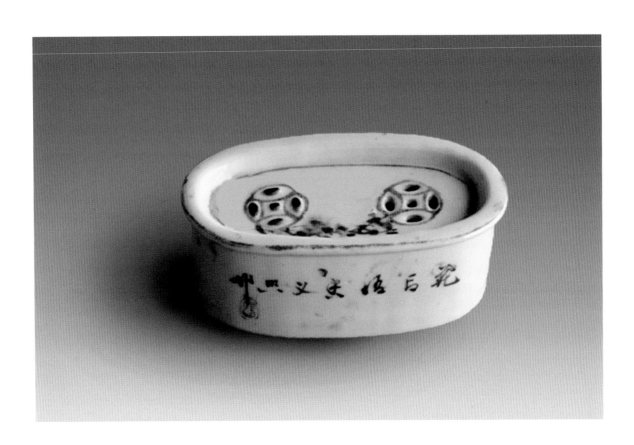

皂盒

民国时期

瓷质

长 12 厘米，宽 6.5 厘米，高 4.5 厘米

Soapbox

Republican Period

Porcelain

Length 12 cm/ Width 6.5 cm/ Height 4.5 cm

长方椭圆形，直口平底圈足，外底部有"李义兴造"朱色铭，饰彩色花鸟纹，盖内凹与器身相扣，上饰彩色花卉及两个镂空的圆形万字孔。由四川省文物总店征集。

成都中医药大学中医药传统文化博物馆藏

The rectangular and oval soapbox has a straight mouth, a flat bottom and a ring foot. The exterior bottom has inscriptions "Made by Li Yixing" painted in red color and is decorated with the patterns of colorful flowers and birds. The lid concaves downward and buckles the body tightly. The whole box is decorated with colorful flowers and plants and two round engraving holes of swastika designs. This item was collected from Sichuan Provincial Cultural Relics Store.

Preserved in Museum of Traditional Chinese Medicine Culture, Chengdu University of Traditional Chinese Medicine

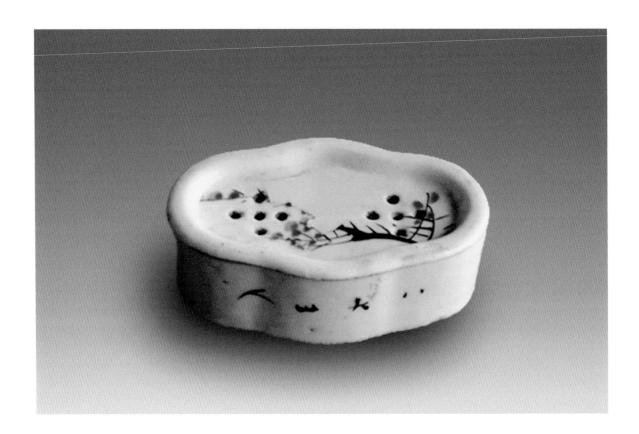

皂盒

民国时期

瓷质

长 10 厘米，宽 6.5 厘米，高 3 厘米

Soapbox

Republican Period

Porcelain

Length 10 cm/ Width 6.5 cm/ Height 3 cm

长方瓜棱形，器身饰有彩色花鸟纹和"八大山
人"墨字，盖内凹与器身相扣，上绘花卉纹，
有两组各五个小圆孔。由四川省文物总店征集。

成都中医药大学中医药传统文化博物馆藏

The soapbox is a rectangular and melon
prismatic shape. It is decorated with the
patterns of colorful flowers and birds and some
Chinese characters "Ba Da Shan Ren" in ink.
The lid concaves downward and buckles the
body tightly. The whole box is decorated
with colorful flowers and plants and has two
sets of small round holes, with five for each
set. This item was collected from Sichuan
Provincial Cultural Relics Store.

Preserved in Museum of Traditional Chinese
Medicine Culture, Chengdu University of
Traditional Chinese Medicine

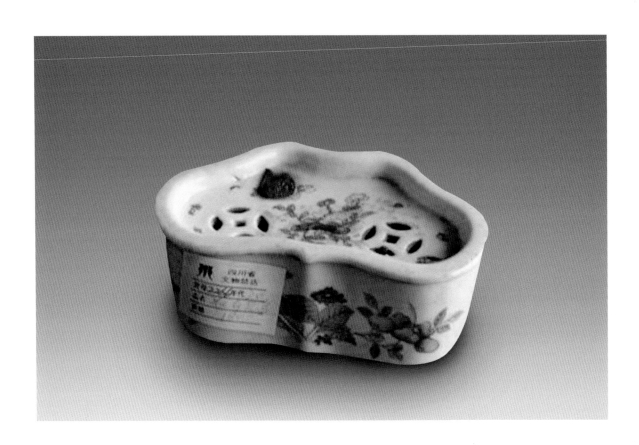

皂盒

民国时期

瓷质

长 12 厘米，宽 7.5 厘米，高 4 厘米

Soapbox

Republican Period

Porcelain

Length 12 cm/ Width 7.5 cm/ Height 4 cm

长方瓜棱形，平口直腹圈足，足底有"江西义成公司"铭，器身饰彩色花卉人物纹和"春色宜人"等文字，盖下凹与器身形成扣口，上饰花卉纹和两个镂空的圆形万字孔。由四川省文物总店征集。

成都中医药大学中医药传统文化博物馆藏

The soapbox is a rectangular and melon prismatic shape. It has a straight mouth, a straight belly and a ring foot on which are painted with inscriptions "Made by Yicheng Company in Jiangxi Province". The body is decorated with colorful flowers and plants and some Chinese characters "Chun Se Yi Ren", meaning the beautiful scenery. The lid concaves downward and buckles the body tightly. The whole box is decorated with colorful flowers and plants and two round engraving holes of swastika designs. This item was collected from Sichuan Provincial Cultural Relics Store.

Preserved in Museum of Traditional Chinese Medicine Culture, Chengdu University of Traditional Chinese Medicine

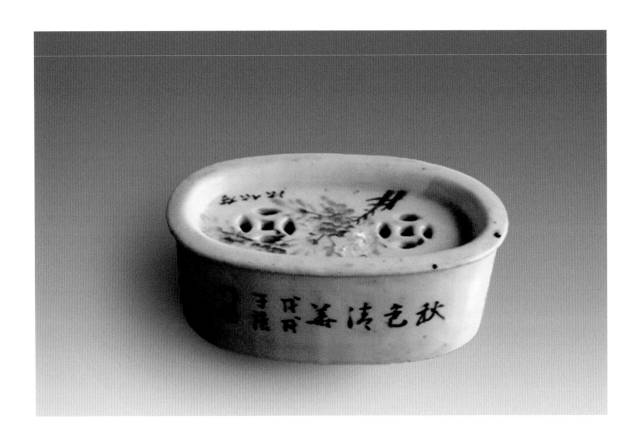

皂盒

民国时期

瓷质

长 11.5 厘米，宽 6.5 厘米，高 4.5 厘米

Soapbox

Republican Period

Porcelain

Length 11.5 cm/ Width 6.5 cm/ Height 4.5 cm

长方椭圆形，平口，直腹，圈足，盖下凹，与器身形成扣口，盖上有彩色树枝纹饰和两个镂空的圆形万字孔，器身饰五彩花鸟纹，并墨书"秋色清义"等纹，为盛放皂胰之用具。由四川省文物总店征集。

成都中医药大学中医药传统文化博物馆藏

The soapbox is a rectangular and oval shape. It has a plain top, a straight belly and a ring foot. The lid concaves downward and buckles the body tightly. The lid is decorated with the patterns of colorful twigs and two round engraving holes of swastika designs. The body is decorated with the patterns of multicolored flowers and birds together with some Chinese characters "Qiu Se Qing Yi". This item, which was utilized for storing soap, was collected from Sichuan Provincial Cultural Relics Store.

Preserved in Museum of Traditional Chinese Medicine Culture, Chengdu University of Traditional Chinese Medicine

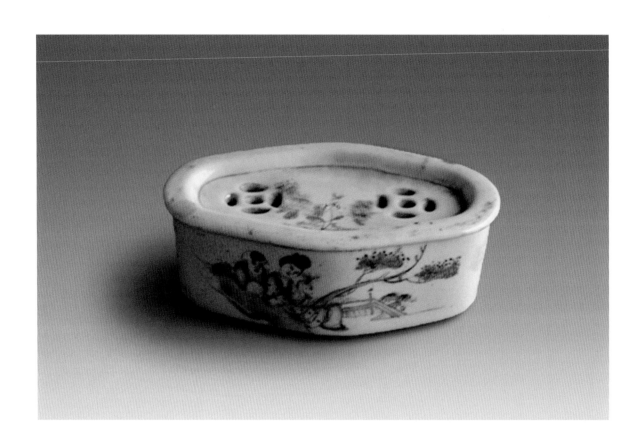

皂盒

民国时期

瓷质

长 9 厘米

Soapbox

Republican Period

Porcelain

Length 9 cm

菱形，平口，直腹，器身饰彩绘母女游玩图，盖下凹与器身形成扣口，上饰花卉纹和两个镂空的圆形万字孔。由四川省文物总店征集。

成都中医药大学中医药传统文化博物馆藏

The soapbox is in the shape of diamond and has a flat mouth and a straight belly. The body of the box is decorated with colorful figures of a mother and her daughter strolling about. The concave cover is decorated with the designs of flowers and two hollow round holes and forms a buckle mouth with the box body. The box was collected from Sichuan Provincial Cultural Relics Store.

Preserved in Museum of Traditional Chinese Medicine Culture, Chengdu University of Traditional Chinese Medicine

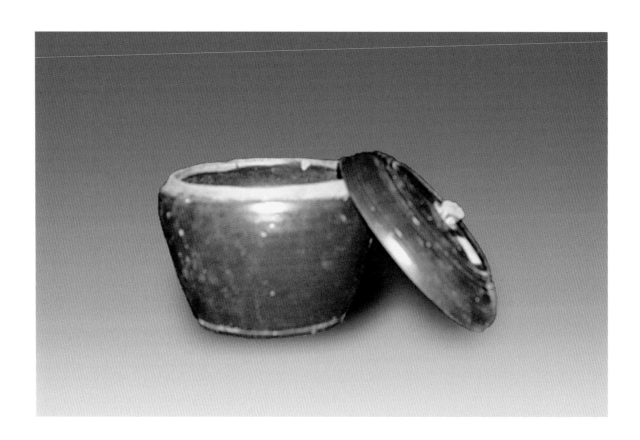

带盖瓷盒

近代

瓷质

口径 15.5 厘米，底径 11.5 厘米，通高 16 厘米，重 1250 克

Porcelain Jar with Lid

Modern Times

Porcelain

Mouth Diameter 15.5 cm/ Foot Diameter 11.5 cm/ Height 16 cm/ Weight 1250 g

子母口，斜腹，圈足，带盖，棕色釉。盛贮器，
完整无损。

陕西医史博物馆藏

With two matching mouths, the jar has an oblique
belly, a ring foot and a lid. The entire jar is covered
with brown glaze. This item, which was utilized
for storing, is still in good condition.

Preserved in Shaanxi Museum of Medical History

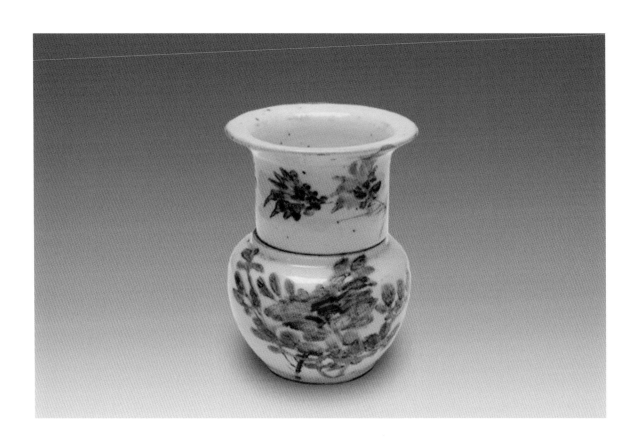

唾盂

民国时期

瓷质

底径 8 厘米，高 10 厘米

Spittoon

Republican Period

Porcelain

Bottom Diameter 8 cm/ Height 10 cm

上、下两层，上部为直筒形，口微敞，下部
为鼓形，浅圈足底，底有"江子钰造"朱砂
铭文。器身饰彩色花鸟纹饰。由民间征集。

成都中医药大学中医药传统文化博物馆藏

The spittoon consists of upper and lower
layers. The upper part is a straight barrel
shape with a slightly flared mouth, while
the lower part is bulgy with a shallow ring
foot. Inscriptions "Made by Jiang Ziyu"
in cinnabar are painted at the bottom. The
entire surface is decorated with the patterns
of colorful birds and flowers. This item was
collected from a private owner.

Preserved in Museum of Traditional Chinese
Medicine Culture, Chengdu University of
Traditional Chinese Medicine

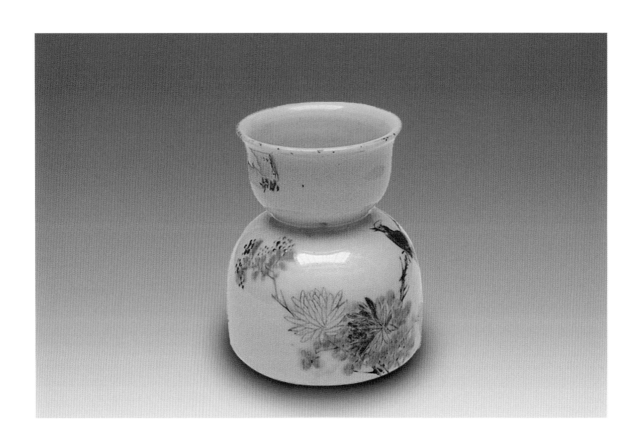

唾盂

清末

瓷质

口径 6.5 厘米，底径 8.4 厘米，高 9.3 厘米

Spittoon

Late Qing Dynasty

Porcelain

Mouth Diameter 6.5 cm/ Bottom Diameter 8.4 cm/ Height 9.3 cm

上、下两层连在一起，且上边较小，底部较大，摆放平稳。上饰彩色花鸟纹饰，底部有"官窑内造"朱砂铭文。由民间征集。

成都中医药大学中医药传统文化博物馆藏

The smaller top and the bigger bottom of the spittoon are connected together. The surface is covered with the patterns of colorful flowers and birds and there is an inscription "Made in Official Kiln" in cinnabar painted at the bottom. This item was collected from a private owner.

Preserved in Museum of Traditional Chinese Medicine Culture, Chengdu University of Traditional Chinese Medicine

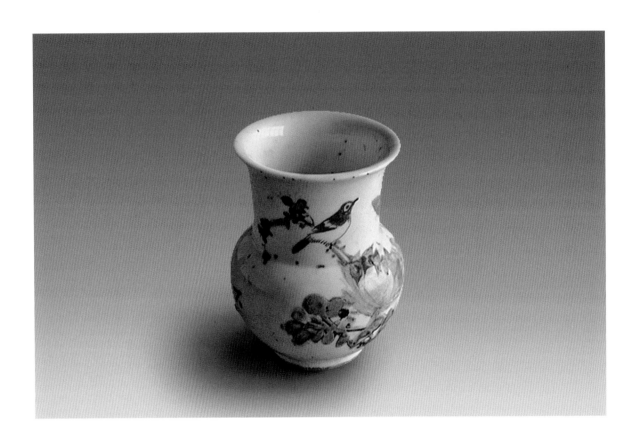

唾盂

民国时期

瓷质

口径 7 厘米，高 10 厘米

Spittoon

Republican Period

Porcelain

Mouth Diameter 7 cm/ Height 10 cm

敞口，直肩，鼓腹，圈足，足底有朱色"景镇陶官窑造"铭，饰彩色花鸟纹。由民间征集。

成都中医药大学中医药传统文化博物馆藏

The spittoon has a flared opening, a straight shoulder, a bulgy belly and a ring foot. At the bottom is the red inscription "Made in Official Porcelain Kiln in Jingdezhen". The item is decorated with the patterns of colorful flowers and birds. The spittoon was collected from a private owner.

Preserved in Museum of Traditional Chinese Medicine Culture, Chengdu University of Traditional Chinese Medicine

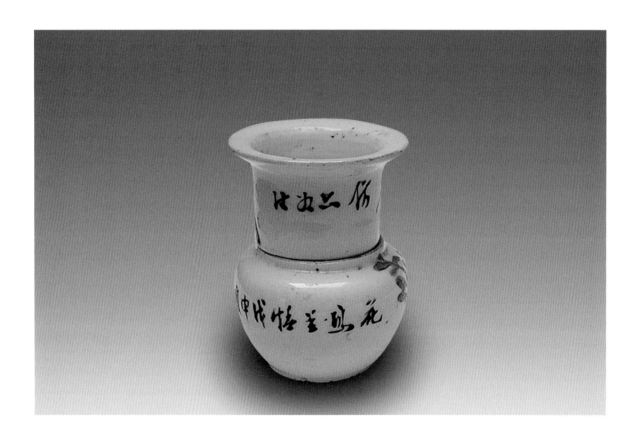

唾盂

民国时期

瓷质

底径 8 厘米，高 10 厘米

Spittoon

Republican Period

Porcelain

Bottom Diameter 8 cm/ Height 10 cm

上、下两层，上部为直筒形，口微敞，下部为鼓形，浅圈足底，底有"江子钰造"朱砂铭文。器形饰彩色花鸟纹饰。由民间征集。

成都中医药大学中医药传统文化博物馆藏

The spittoon consists of upper and lower layers. The upper part is a straight barrel shape with a slightly flared mouth, while the lower part is bulgy with a shallow ring foot. Inscriptions "Made by Jiang Ziyu" in cinnabar are painted at the bottom. The entire surface is decorated with the patterns of colorful birds and flowers. This item was collected from a private owner.

Preserved in Museum of Traditional Chinese Medicine Culture, Chengdu University of Traditional Chinese Medicine

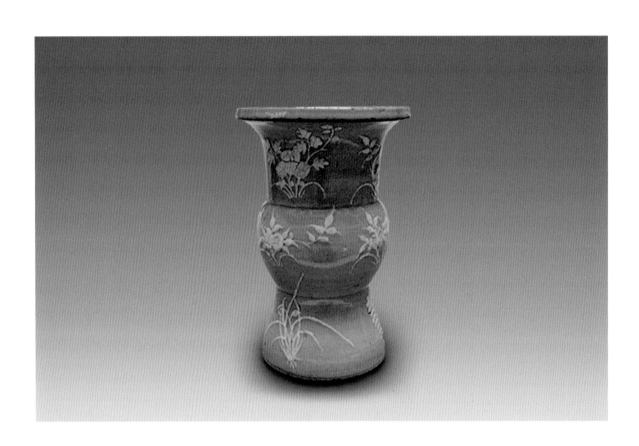

高足痰盂

近代

瓷质

口径 21.5 厘米，高 32.58 厘米

High-foot Spittoon

Modern Times

Porcelain

Mouth Diameter 21.5 cm/ Height 32.58 cm

鼓腹，平底，敞口足，足底有露胎痕迹，直颈，口微敞，口沿直立，器身贴塑花草纹饰，施豆青釉，色泽莹润，器形完整，是晚清以后常见的放置于地面的吐痰用具，大多摆放在客厅等待客之处。由四川省文物总店征集。

成都中医药大学中医药传统文化博物馆藏

The spittoon has a bulgy belly, a flat bottom and an open foot. There is uncovered base color at the bottom of the foot. The spittoon has a straight neck and a slight open mouth and a vertical mouth rim. The body is decorated with the patterns of flowers and grass in celadon glaze. Bright and smooth in color and intact in shape, this item was a common spittoon placed on the ground in the late Qing Dynasty and was mostly found in the living room or other reception places. It was collected from Sichuan Provincial Cultural Relics Store.

Preserved in Museum of Traditional Chinese Medicine Culture, Chengdu University of Traditional Chinese Medicine

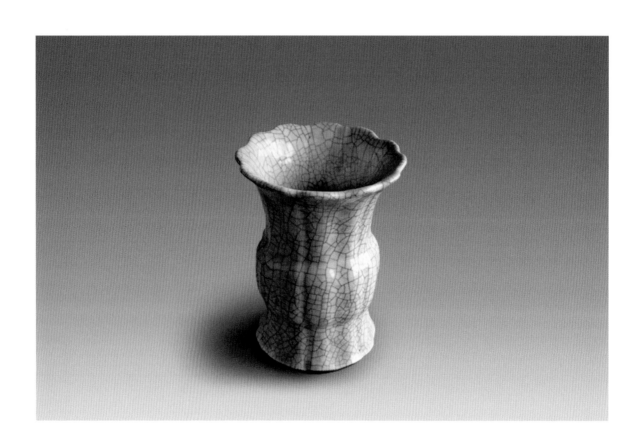

唾盂

民国时期

瓷质

口径 18.5 厘米，底径 14.5 厘米，高 24 厘米

Spittoon

Republican Period

Porcelain

Mouth Diameter 18.5 cm/ Bottom Diameter 14.5 cm/ Height 24 cm

仿哥窑冰裂纹，青色釉，器身为瓜棱形，口部呈葵瓣形，器形较大，多用于客厅或其他公共场合。由上海文物总店征集。

成都中医药大学中医药传统文化博物馆藏

The spittoon has the ice crack patterns made by imitation of Ge Kiln in celadon glaze. The ware is a rectangular and melon prismatic shape. The mouth is shaped like a sunflower petal. With a big size, this kind of ware was frequently utilized in the living room or other public places. It was collected from Shanghai Cultural Relics Store.

Preserved in Museum of Traditional Chinese Medicine Culture, Chengdu University of Traditional Chinese Medicine

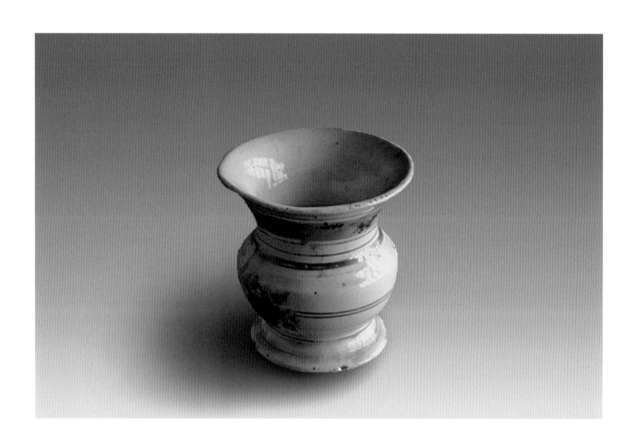

唾盂

民国时期

瓷质

口径 7.8 厘米，高 7.6 厘米

Spittoon

Republican Period

Porcelain

Mouth Diameter 7.8 cm/ Height 7.6 cm

敞口，彭腹，圈足，腹部贴有花卉纹饰，颈部及肩部贴有金色带状纹，是小巧精致的吐痰用具。由四川省文物总店征集。

成都中医药大学中医药传统文化博物馆藏

The spittoon has a flared mouth, a bulgy belly and a ring foot. With flower decorations on the belly and golden strip designs on the neck and shoulder, this item is a small but delicate spittoon. It was collected from Sichuan Provincial Cultural Relics Store.

Preserved in Museum of Traditional Chinese Medicine Culture, Chengdu University of Traditional Chinese Medicine

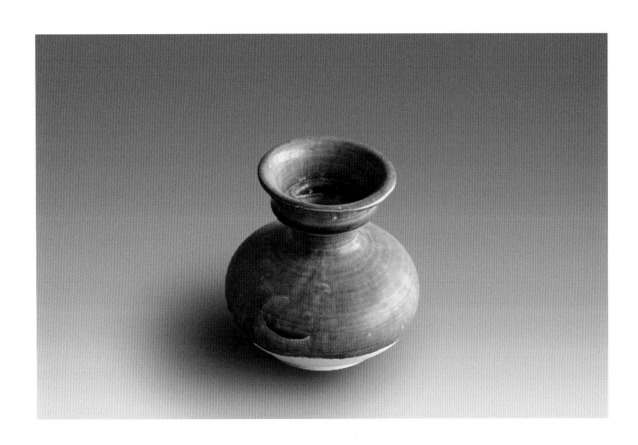

唾盂

近代

瓷质

口径 7.5 厘米，高 10 厘米

Spittoon

Modern Times

Porcelain

Mouth Diameter 7.5 cm/ Height 10 cm

敞口，鼓腹，平底，大部分施青釉，底部露胎。
由民间征集。

成都中医药大学中医药传统文化博物馆藏

The spittoon has a flared opening, a bulgy belly and a flat bottom. Most parts are in celadon glaze and the bottom is uncovered base color. It was collected from a private owner.

Preserved in Museum of Traditional Chinese Medicine Culture, Chengdu University of Traditional Chinese Medicine

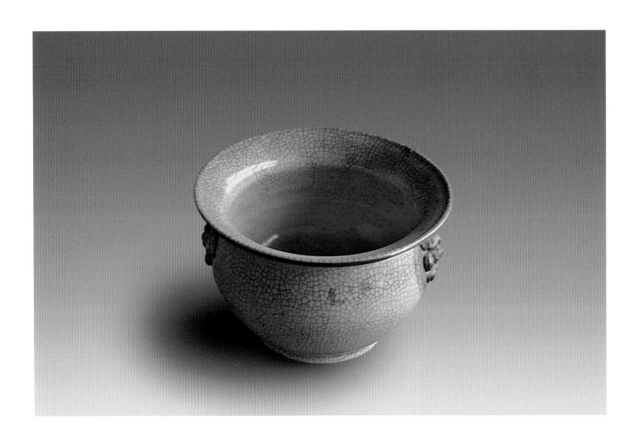

香炉

近代

瓷质

口径 16.5 厘米，高 10.5 厘米

Censer

Modern Times

Porcelain

Mouth Diameter 16.5 cm/ Height 10.5 cm

敞口，束颈，鼓腹，圈足，肩部有三个堆塑的兽形装饰，通体施青釉，上有冰裂纹。由民间征集。

成都中医药大学中医药传统文化博物馆藏

This censer has a flared mouth, a contracting neck, a bulgy belly and a ring foot. There are three paste-on-paste decorations of beasts on the shoulder. With ice crack patterns on it, the entire ware is covered with celadon glaze. The Censer was collected from a private owner.

Preserved in Museum of Traditional Chinese Medicine Culture, Chengdu University of Traditional Chinese Medicine

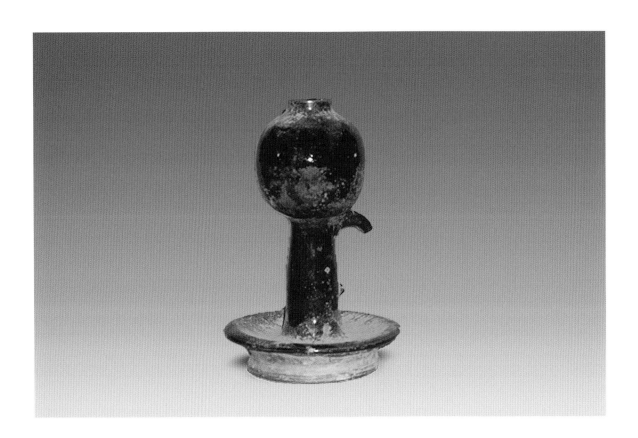

黑釉灯

近代

瓷质

口径 2.9 厘米，底径 8.6 厘米，高 17 厘米，重 700 克

Black Glazed Oil Lamp

Modern Times

Porcelain

Mouth Diameter 2.9 cm/ Bottom Diameter 8.6 cm/ Height 17 cm/ Weight 700 g

直口,圆腹,圆柄带一耳,盘座,浅圈足,通体黑釉,圈足无釉。生活用器。有残。1999 年 12 月 8 日入藏,陕西省澄城县征集。

陕西医史博物馆藏

This item has a straight mouth, a round belly, a round handle with an ear, a round stand and a shallow ring foot. The entire body is covered with black glaze with the exception of the ring foot. This daily utensil is slightly damaged. It was collected from Chengcheng County, Shaanxi Province, on December 8th, 1999.

Preserved in Shaanxi Museum of Medical History

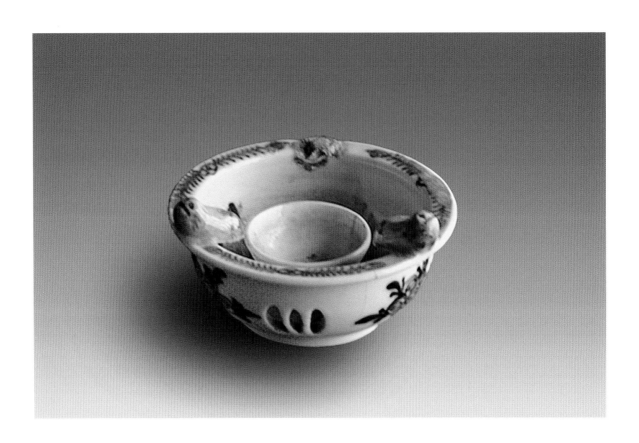

灯

民国时期

瓷质

口径 9.5 厘米，高 4 厘米

Oil Lamp

Republican Period

Porcelain

Mouth Diameter 9.5 cm/ Height 4 cm

内、外两层，可减少灯油的损耗，外壁施青
花草叶纹饰。由民间征集。

　　成都中医药大学中医药传统文化博物馆藏

The lamp has internal and external layers.
These two layers can reduce the loss of the
lamp oil. The exterior wall of the lamp is
decorated with the patterns of blue-and-white
leaves of grass. The lamp was collected from
a private owner.

Preserved in Museum of Traditional Chinese
Medicine Culture, Chengdu University of
Traditional Chinese Medicine

粉彩花虫纹印盒

近代

瓷质

口径 6.4 厘米，高 2.5 厘米

Famille-rose Seal Box Painted with Designs of Flowers and Insects

Modern Times

Porcelain

Mouth Diameter 6.4 cm/ Height 2.5 cm

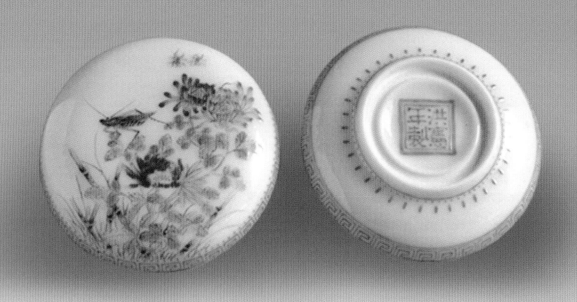

盖面彩绘花卉、草蜢、蜜蜂等纹饰，底用蓝料书写"洪宪年制"四字双方框款。色彩鲜艳，白釉莹润，绘画工艺精致，草虫栩栩如生。

卢晓晖藏

The box is painted with the designs of color drawings and plants, grasshoppers, bees and so on. The seal is in the shape of double square frames with four Chinese characters inside, meaning "Made in the Year of Hongxian". Bright color, smooth white and exquisite painting techniques make the pictures vivid and lifelike.

Preserved by Lu Xiaohui

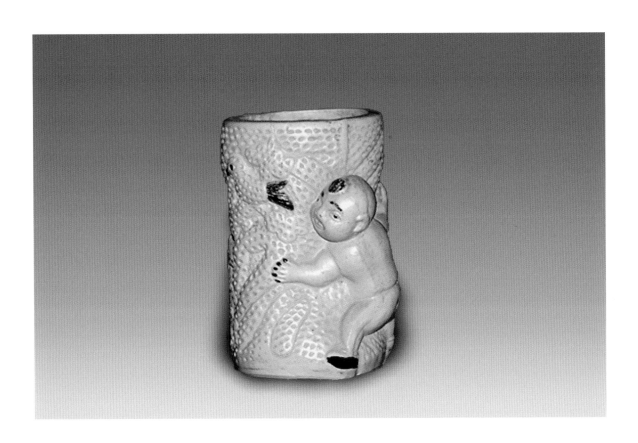

笔筒

近代

瓷质

口径 6.2 厘米，底径 6.2 厘米，通高 9.5 厘米，重 150 克

Brush Holder

Modern Times

Porcelain

Mouth Diameter 6.2 cm/ Bottom Diameter 6.2 cm/ Height 9.5 cm/ Weight 150 g

直口,直腹,平底,笔筒上有浮雕,底有"左光""造"
字样。文房四宝,完整无损。陕西省西安市征集。

陕西医史博物馆藏

The brush holder is straight from the mouth to the belly, with a flat bottom. Carvings in relief are found on the brush pot and Chinese characters "Zuoguang" and "Zao" are at the bottom. It is one of the four treasures of study and is still in good condition. The brush holder was collected in Xi'an, Shaanxi Province.

Preserved in Shaanxi Museum of Medical History

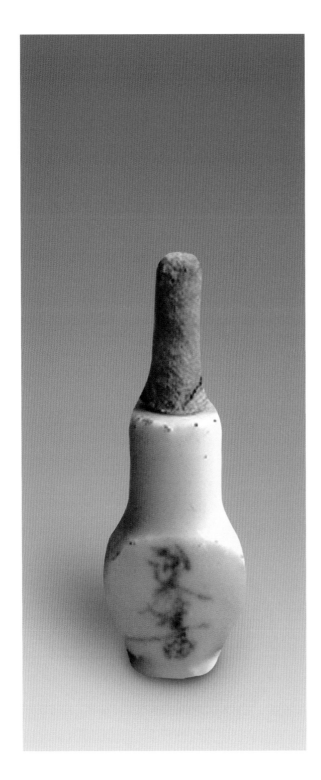

瓷鼻烟壶

近代

瓷质

口径 0.8 厘米，腹宽 2 厘米，高 3.8 厘米

Porcelain Snuff Bottle

Modern Times

Porcelain

Mouth Diameter 0.8 cm/ Belly Diameter 2 cm/

Height 3.8 cm

扁圆形，直口，长颈，溜肩，平底。小药瓶，
上有塞子。

江苏省中医药博物馆藏

This ware is a small medicine bottle with a
stopper on it. The oblate bottle has a straight
mouth, a long neck, a smooth shoulder and a
flat bottom.
Preserved in Jiangsu Museum of Traditional
Chinese Medicine

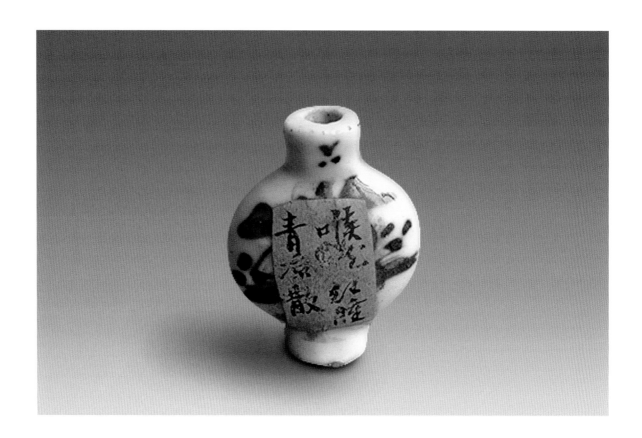

瓷鼻烟壶

近代

瓷质

口径 0.7 厘米，腹宽 4 厘米，高 5.4 厘米

Porcelain Snuff Bottle

Modern Times

Porcelain

Mouth Diameter 0.7 cm/ Belly Diameter 4 cm/ Height 5.4 cm

塑像连底座。孙思邈，唐朝著名医学家，著《千
金方》，对药物有深入研究，后世尊称其为药王。
此塑像为现代制，为纪念孙氏对医学的伟大贡献。

广东中医药博物馆藏

The porcelain. statue joins its pedestal Sun Simiao,
a famous medical expert in the Tang Dynasty,
wrote a book named "Qian Jin Fang" (*Thousand
Golden Prescriptions*). His profound research in
drugs and medicine earned him the title, the King of
Medicine. This statue was made in modern times to
commemorate his contributions to medicine.

Preserved in Guangdong Chinese Medicine Museum

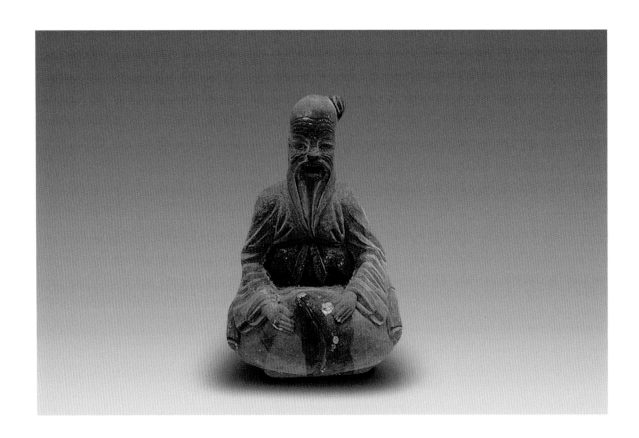

寿星

民国时期

灰塑

高 49 厘米

Statue of the God of Longevity

Republican Period

Clay

Height 49 cm

衣服部位有彩色装饰，表达人们期望长寿的
美好祝福。由民间征集。

成都中医药大学中医药传统文化博物馆藏

Colorful decorations can be found in some
parts of the clothes. This statue conveys
people's best wishes for longevity. It was
collected from a private owner.
Preserved in Museum of Traditional Chinese
Medicine Culture, Chengdu University of
Traditional Chinese Medicine

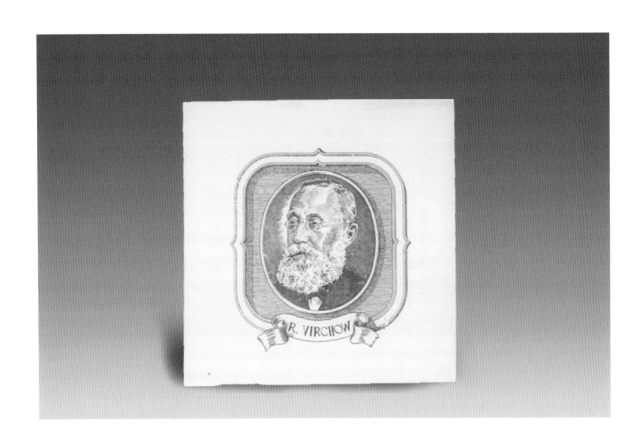

瓷板人物画

近现代

瓷质

长 15 厘米，宽 15 厘米

Vitrolite Figure Painting

Modern Times

Porcelain

Length 15 cm/ Width 15 cm

方形，为艺术品。该藏品以白方瓷砖为底
板，上绿釉绘有"R. VIRCHOW"的人头像，
制作精细。外面封套上印有"拜耳药品无
限公司谨赠"字样，保存基本完好。1955
年入藏。

中华医学会 / 上海中医药博物馆藏

This delicate work of art is square with
a white porcelain plate as its base, on
which the head portrait of R. VIRCHOW is
painted in green glaze. The words printed on
the outside of the plate cover means "with
the compliments of Bayer Pharmaceutical
Company Unlimited". The plate is still in
good condition. It was collected in 1955.
Preserved in Chinese Medical Association/
Museum of Chinese Medicine, Shanghai
University of Traditional Chinese Medicine

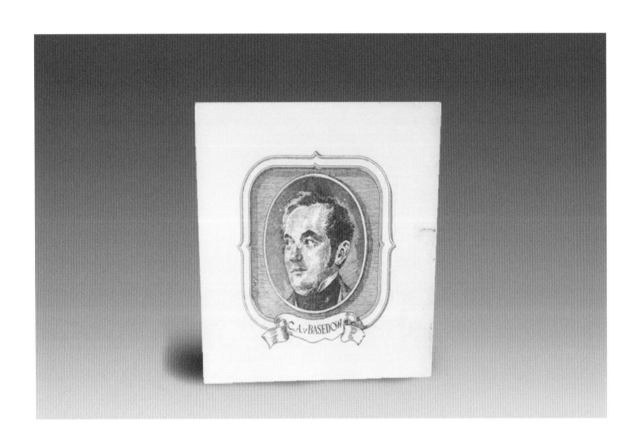

瓷板人物画

近现代

瓷质

长 15 厘米，宽 15 厘米

Vitrolite Figure Painting

Modern Times

Porcelain

Length 15 cm/ Width 15 cm

方形，为艺术品。该藏品以白方瓷砖为底
板，上绿釉绘有"C.A.V BASEDOW"的
人头像，制作精细。外面封套上印有"拜
耳药品无限公司谨赠"字样，保存基本完
好。1955 年入藏。

中华医学会 / 上海中医药博物馆藏

This delicate work of art is square with a
white porcelain plate as its base, on which
the head portrait of C.A.V BASEDOW is
painted in green glaze. The words printed
on the outside of the plate cover means "with
the compliments of Bayer Pharmaceutical
Company Unlimited". The plate is still in
good condition. It was collected in 1955.
Preserved in Chinese Medical Association/
Museum of Chinese Medicine, Shanghai
University of Traditional Chinese Medicine

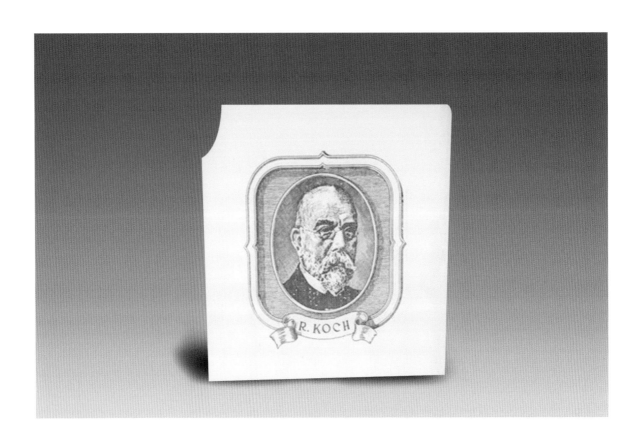

瓷板人物画

近现代

瓷质

长 15 厘米，宽 15 厘米

Vitrolite Figure Painting

Modern Times

Porcelain

Length 15 cm/ Width 15 cm

方形，为艺术品。该藏品以白方瓷砖为底板，上绿釉绘有"R. KOCH"的人头像，制作精细。外面封套上印有"拜耳药品无限公司谨赠"字样。1955 年入藏。

中华医学会 / 上海中医药博物馆藏

This delicate work of art is square with a white porcelain plate as its base, on which the head portrait of R. KOCH is painted in green glaze. The words printed on the outside of the plate cover means "with the compliments of Bayer Pharmaceutical Company Unlimited". It was collected in 1955.

Preserved in Chinese Medical Association/ Museum of Chinese Medicine, Shanghai University of Traditional Chinese Medicine

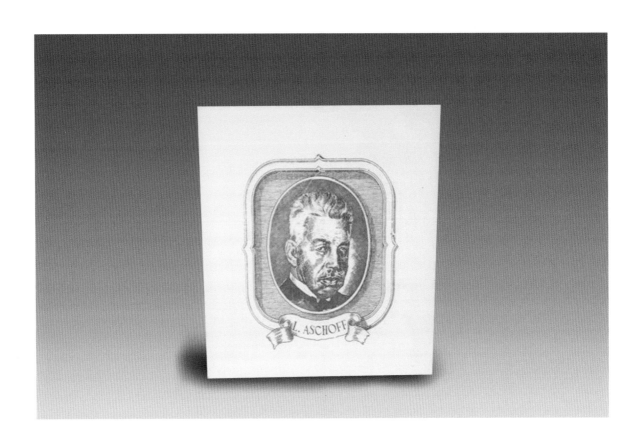

瓷板人物画

近现代

瓷质

长 15 厘米，宽 15 厘米

Vitrolite Figure Painting

Modern Times

Porcelain

Length 15 cm/ Width 15 cm

方形，为艺术品。该藏品以白方瓷砖为底板，上绿釉绘有"L. ASCHOFF"的人头像，制作精细。外面封套上印有"拜耳药品无限公司谨赠"字样，保存基本完好。1955年入藏。

中华医学会 / 上海中医药博物馆藏

This delicate work of art is square with a white porcelain plate as its base, on which the head portrait of L. ASCHOFF is painted in green glaze. The words printed on the outside of the plate cover means "with the compliments of Bayer Pharmaceutical Company Unlimited". The plate is still in good condition. It was collected in 1955.

Preserved in Chinese Medical Association/ Museum of Chinese Medicine, Shanghai University of Traditional Chinese Medicine

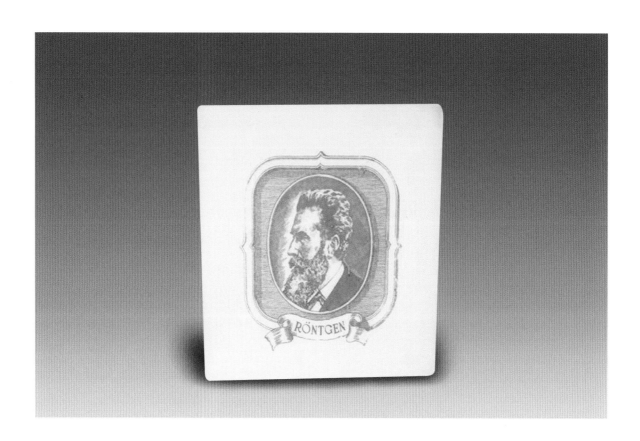

瓷板人物画

近现代

瓷质

长 15 厘米，宽 15 厘米

Vitrolite Figure Painting

Modern Times

Porcelain

Length 15 cm/ Width 15 cm

方形，为艺术品。该藏品以白方瓷砖为底板，上绿釉绘有"RONTGEN"的人头像，制作精细。外面封套上印有"拜耳药品无限公司谨赠"字样，保存基本完好。1955年入藏。

中华医学会 / 上海中医药博物馆藏

This delicate work of art is square with a white porcelain plate as its base, on which the head portrait of RONTGEN is painted in green glaze. The words printed on the outside of the plate cover means "with the compliments of Bayer Pharmaceutical Company Unlimited". The plate is still in good condition. It was collected in 1955.

Preserved in Chinese Medical Association/ Museum of Chinese Medicine, Shanghai University of Traditional Chinese Medicine

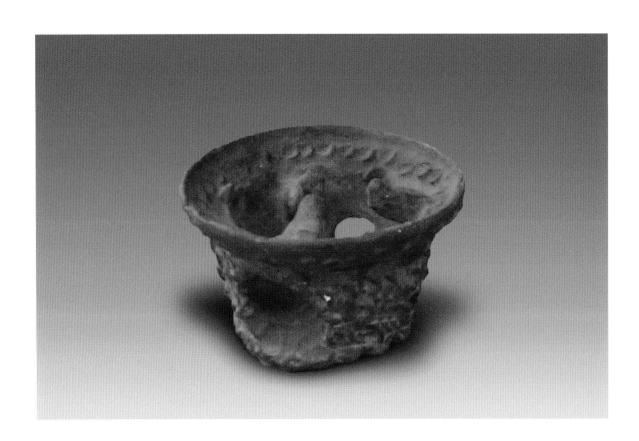

陶灶

近现代

红砂陶

口径 18.5 厘米，底径 12.4 厘米，通高 11.3 厘米

Pottery Stove

Modern Times

Red Pottery Sand

Mouth Diameter 18.5 cm/ Bottom Diameter 12.4 cm/ Height 11.3 cm

仿汉现代复制品，圆盆状，平底，敞口，
炉膛内有三个支脚，灶身近底部有两灶口，
工艺粗糙。保存基本完好，为明器复制品。

中华医学会 / 上海中医药博物馆藏

This round basin-shaped Han-style replica
of pottery stove is made of red pottery
sand. It is flat-bottomed and has an open
mouth. The stove has three feet and two
mouths near the bottom of the stove. It
is rough in craftwork. As the replica of a
funerary ware, the stove is still in good
condition.

Preserved in Chinese Medical Association/
Museum of Chinese Medicine, Shanghai
University of Traditional Chinese Medicine

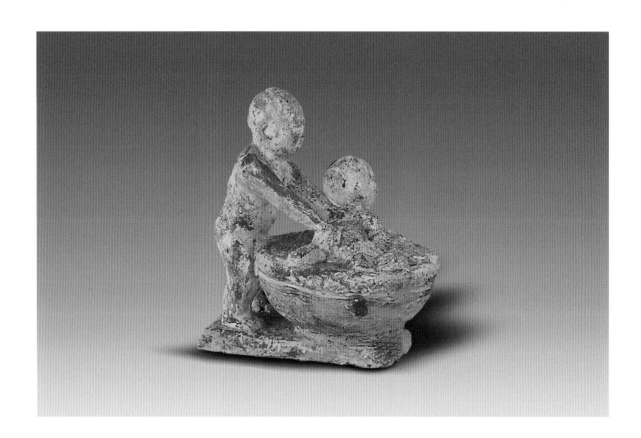

陶洗澡俑

现代

陶质

Pottery Bathing Figurine

Modern Times

Pottery

不规则形，明器。该藏为仿唐复制品，灰
陶制成，为一成人给幼儿于盆内洗澡，形
象生动，造型美观。1955 年入藏。保存
基本完好。

中华医学会 / 上海中医药博物馆藏

This irregularly shaped Tang-style pottery
bathing figurine is a funerary ware made
of gray pottery. It is vivid and attractive. It
is made like an adult bathing a child in the
basin. Collected in 1955, the figurine and
is still in good condition.
Preserved in Chinese Medical Association/
Museum of Chinese Medicine, Shanghai
University of Traditional Chinese Medicine

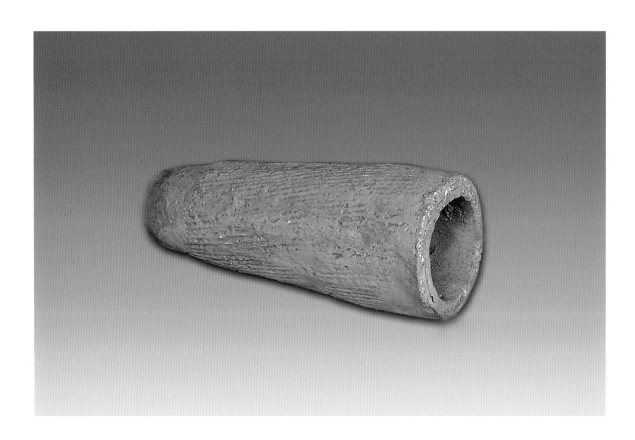

陶水管

现代

陶质

粗径 1.52 厘米，细径 1.02 厘米，通长 42.3 厘米，壁厚 2.15 厘米

Pottery Water Pipe

Modern Times

Pottery

Thick Diameter 1.52 cm/ Thin Diameter 1.02 cm/ Length 42.3 cm/ Thickness of the Wall 2.15 cm

圆管形，为卫生设施水管部件。复制品，灰陶制成，一头粗一头细，表面有长条纹，工艺一般。1955 年入藏。保存基本完好。

中华医学会 / 上海中医药博物馆藏

This tube-shaped replica of pottery water pipe is made of gray pottery. As a part of water pipeline for sanitation facility, it is thick in one end and thin in the other with long stripes on the surface. It is mediocre in craftwork. Collected in 1955, the pipe is still in good condition.

Preserved in Chinese Medical Association/ Museum of Chinese Medicine, Shanghai University of Traditional Chinese Medicine

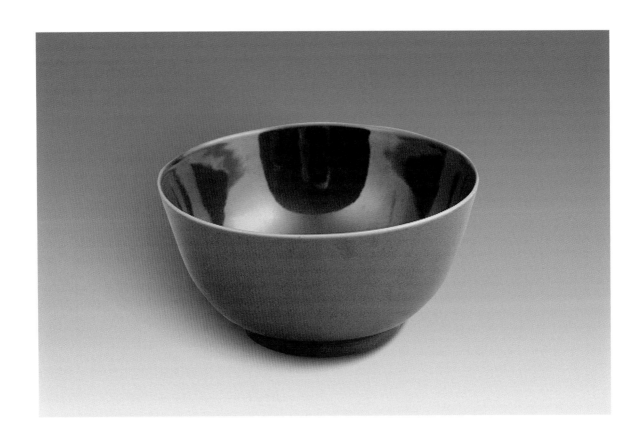

酱釉碗

清

瓷质

直径 12 厘米

Reddish-brown-glazed Bowl

Qing Dynasty

Porcelain

Diameter 12 cm

敞口，平底，圈足。胎质细腻，做工精致，官窑出品。皇帝用于喝中药的碗，酱釉颜色和中药汤颜色相近，有利于缓解生病喝药时的紧张情绪。

北京御生堂中医药博物馆藏

The bowl has a flared mouth, a flat bottom and a ring foot. The porcelain body is fine and smooth with exquisite workmanship, and is the product of official kiln. It was a bowl used by emperors to take Chinese medicine. The color of reddish brown is close to that of the traditional Chinese medicine soup, which could lessen the patients' anxiety when taking the medicine.

Preserved in Chinese Medicine Museum of Beijing Yu Sheng Tang Drugstore

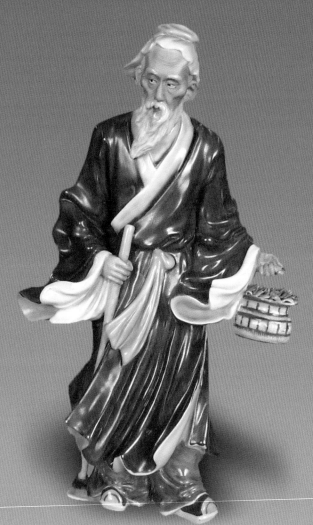

扁鹊瓷像

近现代

瓷质

宽 20 厘米，厚 8.5 厘米，通高 32.8 厘米

Porcelain Figurine of Bian Que

Modern Times

Porcelain

Width 20 cm/ Thickness 8.5 cm/ Height 32.8 cm

人像形，工艺品。该工艺品中扁鹊身着棕褐色长袍，头戴蓝色布帽，右手握锄头，左手提一竹篮，形象逼真。1958 年入藏。有残。

中华医学会 / 上海中医药博物馆藏

This art ware is the portrait of Bian Que (a famous doctor in ancient China). In this vivid porcelain figurine, Bian Que is dressed in a brown robe, wearing a blue cloth hat with a hoe in the right hand and a bamboo basket in the left hand. the incomplete figurine was collected in 1958.

Preserved in Chinese Medical Association/ Museum of Chinese Medicine, Shanghai University of Traditional Chinese Medicine

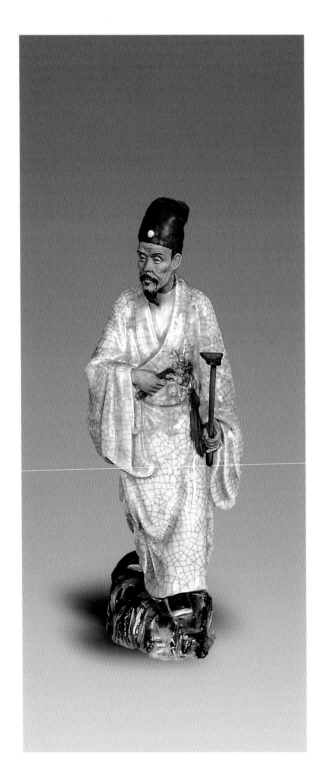

李时珍瓷像

近现代

瓷质

宽 14 厘米，通高 38 厘米

Porcelain Figurine of Li Shizhen

Modern Times

Porcelain

Width 14 cm/ Height 38 cm

人像形，工艺品。该藏施素彩釉，开片，为李时珍奔波于山间采药的形象，其左手持锄，右手握一草药，造型生动。1955 年入藏。保存完好。

中华医学会／上海中医药博物馆藏

This art ware is the portrait of Li Shizhen, a famous doctor in ancient China. This porcelain figurine is covered with cracked plain colored glaze. In this vivid porcelain portrait, Li Shizhen is walking back and forth to collect Chinese medicinal herbs in the mountain with his left hand holding a hoe and his right hand gripping herbal medicine. The figurine was collected in 1955. It is still in good condition.

Preserved in Chinese Medical Association/ Museum of Chinese Medicine, Shanghai University of Traditional Chinese Medicine

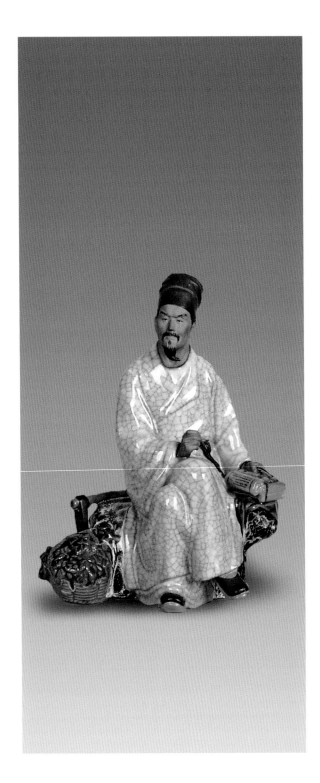

李时珍瓷像

近现代

瓷质

宽 16.8 厘米，通高 22.3 厘米

Porcelain Figurine of Li Shizhen

Modern Times

Porcelain

Width 16.8 cm/ Height 22.3 cm

人像形，工艺品。该藏施彩色釉，开片，为李时珍坐于野外岩石上研究本草的形象，身边有竹篮、锄头和医籍等物。1976年入藏。保存完好。

中华医学会 / 上海中医药博物馆藏

This art ware is the portrait of Li Shizhen, a famous doctor in ancient China. This porcelain figurine is covered with cracked color glaze. In this vivid porcelain portrait, Li Sizhen is sitting on the rocks in the field and studying herbal medicine with bamboo basket, hoe and medical books beside. The figurine was collected in 1976. It is still in good condition.

Preserved in Chinese Medical Association/ Museum of Chinese Medicine, Shanghai University of Traditional Chinese Medicine

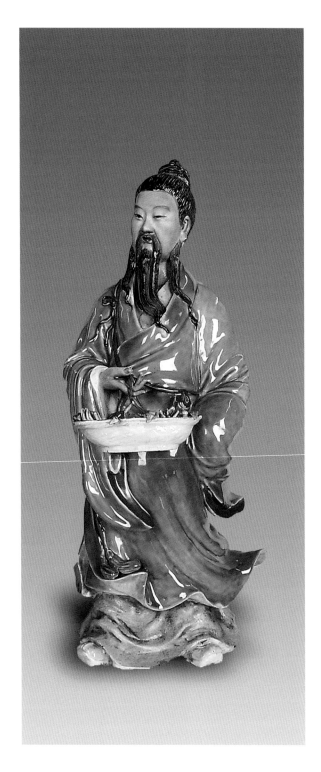

采药人瓷像

近现代

瓷质

宽 17.5 厘米，厚 15 厘米，通高 39.2 厘米

Porcelain Figurine of Herbalist

Modern Times

Porcelain

Width 17.5 cm/ Thickness 15 cm/ Height 39.2 cm

人像形，艺术品。该藏构图为一采药老人身着蓝色长袍，手提黄色篮子，篮中有各种草药。造型生动，工艺一般。1958 年入藏。保存基本完好。

中华医学会 / 上海中医药博物馆藏

This art ware with mediocre craft is the portrait of a herbalist. In this vivid porcelain figurine, an old herbalist dressed in blue robe is holding a yellow basket in the right hand and there are a variety of herbs in the basket. The figurine was collected in 1958. It is still in good condition.

Preserved in Chinese Medical Association/ Museum of Chinese Medicine, Shanghai University of Traditional Chinese Medicine

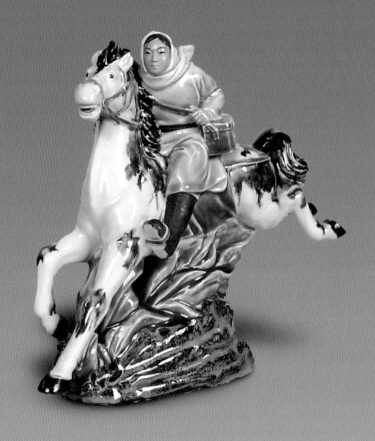

"飞马送医" 瓷塑

近现代

瓷质

宽 26.2 厘米，厚 9 厘米，高 32 厘米

Porcelain Statue of a Doctor on Galloping Horse to Deliver Medicine

Modern Times

Porcelain

Width 26.2 cm/ Thickness 9 cm/ Height 32 cm

人骑马形,艺术品。该藏构图为一草原医生身着草绿长袍,斜挎红十字药箱,骑坐一匹飞奔的白马,送医送药的情景。造型生动,工艺一般。1976 年入藏。保存基本完好。

中华医学会 / 上海中医药博物馆藏

This artwork with mediocre craft is shaped like a man riding a horse. In this vivid porcelain statue, a prairie doctor dressed in grass green robe with a red-cross medical kit slung over the shoulder is riding a white galloping horse to deliver medicine and medical service. The statue was collected in 1976. It is still in good condition. Preserved in Chinese Medical Association/ Museum of Chinese Medicine, Shanghai University of Traditional Chinese Medicine

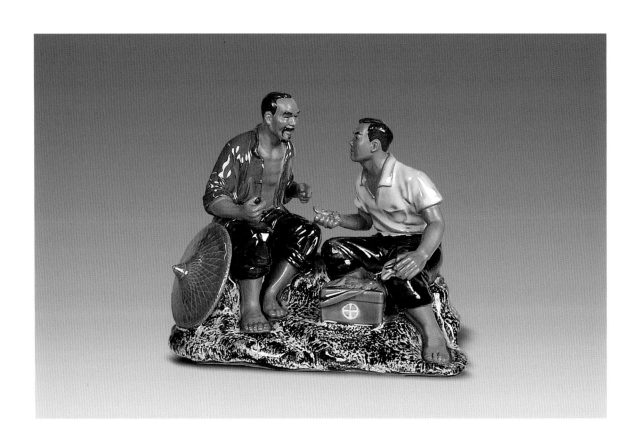

赤脚医生像

现代

瓷质

宽 22.4 厘米，厚 11.8 厘米，通高 19.4 厘米

Figurine of Barefoot Doctors

Modern Times

Porcelain

Width 22.4 cm/ Thickness 11.8 cm/ Height 19.4 cm

人像形，工艺品。该藏施蓝、绿、白各色釉，

为年轻赤脚医生向前辈请教草药知识的形

象。工艺一般。1976 年入藏。保存基本

完好。

中华医学会 / 上海中医药博物馆藏

This art ware with mediocre craft is the

portrait of barefoot doctors. This porcelain

figurine is covered with blue, green and

white colored glaze. In this vivid porcelain

figurine, the young barefoot doctor is

consulting the senior one about herbal

knowledge. The figurine was collected in

1976. It is still in good condition.

Preserved in Chinese Medical Association/

Museum of Chinese Medicine, Shanghai

University of Traditional Chinese Medicine

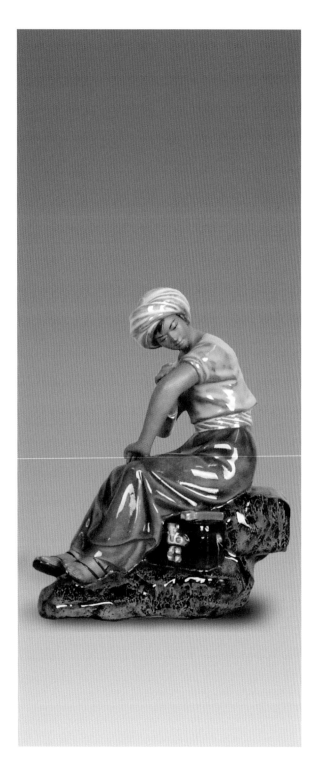

傣族赤脚医生像

现代

瓷质

宽 19 厘米，通高 22.8 厘米

Figurine of Dai Barefoot Doctor

Modern Times

Porcelain

Width 19 cm/ Height 22.8 cm

人像形，工艺品。该藏施蓝、绿、白各色釉，

为傣族赤脚医生在自己身上试针的形象。

工艺一般。1976 年入藏。保存基本完好。

中华医学会 / 上海中医药博物馆藏

This art ware with mediocre craft is the
portrait of Dai barefoot doctors. This
porcelain figurine is covered with blue,
green and white colored glaze. In this vivid
porcelain figurine, the barefoot doctor
of Dai is testing needle on his body. It
was collected in 1976 and is still in good
condition.

Preserved in Chinese Medical Association/
Museum of Chinese Medicine, Shanghai
University of Traditional Chinese Medicine

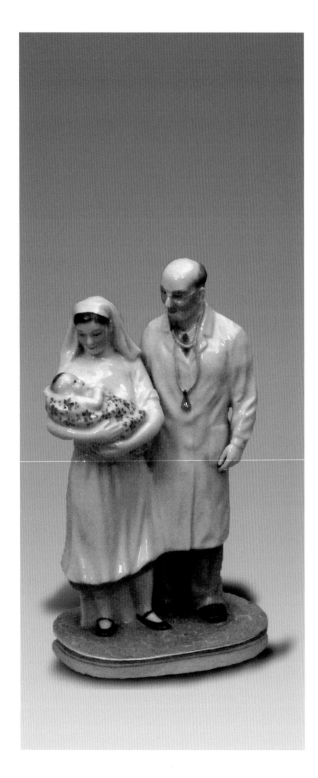

苏联医生和护士瓷像

近现代

瓷质

宽 17.5 厘米，通高 28 厘米

Porcelain Figurine of Doctor and Nurse of Soviet Union

Modern Times

Porcelain

Width 17.5 cm/ Height 28 cm

人像形，工艺品。该藏施白色釉，为一苏
联医生和护士立像，护士怀抱婴儿，头戴
披巾；医生身着白衣，脖戴听诊器。形象
生动，造型美观。1958 年入藏。保存完好。

　　　　中华医学会／上海中医药博物馆藏

This art ware with beautiful appearance is
the Standing Statue of a doctor and a nurse
of Soviet Union. This porcelain figurine is
covered with white colored glaze. In this
vivid porcelain figurine, the Soviet nurse
wearing a shawl is carrying a baby in her
arms, while the Soviet doctor dressed in
white is wearing a stethoscope around his
neck. The Statue was collected in 1958 and
is still in good condition.
Preserved in Chinese Medical Association/
Museum of Chinese Medicine, Shanghai
University of Traditional Chinese Medicine

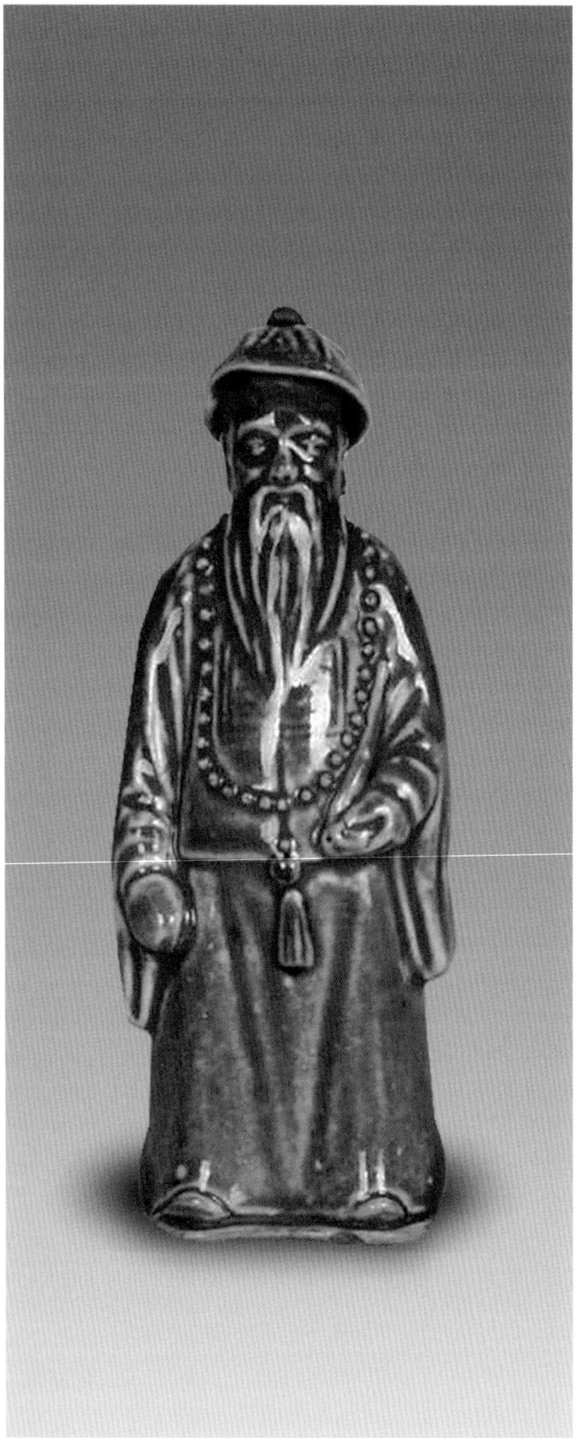

林则徐瓷像

近现代

瓷质

宽 4.6 厘米，厚 3.2 厘米，通高 13.3 厘米

Porcelain Statue of Lin Zexu

Modern Times

Porcelain

Width 4.6 cm/ Thickness 3.2 cm/ Height 13.3 cm

人像形，工艺品。该藏通身施棕褐色釉，
林氏顶戴花翎，身着朝服，后背有长辫。
工艺一般。1961 年入藏。保存完好。

中华医学会 / 上海中医药博物馆藏

The porcelain figure statue is a brown art
work by modest handcraft. The statue of
Lin Zexu, with a long plait at the back, is in
an official hat and a robe. It was collected in
1961 and still in good condition.
Preserved in Chinese Medical Association/
Museum of Chinese Medicine, Shanghai
University of Traditional Chinese Medicine

索 引

（馆藏地按拼音字母排序）

朱德明

Index

Guangdong Chinese Medicine Museum

Jiangsu Museum of Traditional Chinese Medicine

Lu Xiaohui

Shaanxi Museum of Medical History

The Museum of the Republic of China, Shanghai Medical Literature Museum

Private Owner

Tibet Museum

Chinese Medical Association/Museum of Chinese Medicine, Shanghai University of Traditional Chinese Medicine

Zhu Deming

参考文献

[1] 李经纬 . 中国古代医史图录 [M]. 北京：人民卫生出版社，1992.

[2] 傅维康，李经纬，林昭庚 . 中国医学通史：文物图谱卷 [M]. 北京：人民卫生出版社，2000.

[3] 和中浚，吴鸿洲 . 中华医学文物图集 [M]. 成都：四川人民出版社，2001.

[4] 上海中医药博物馆 . 上海中医药博物馆馆藏珍品 [M]. 上海：上海科学技术出版社，2013.

[5] 西藏自治区博物馆 . 西藏博物馆 [M]. 北京：五洲传播出版社，2005.

[6] 崔乐泉 . 中国古代体育文物图录：中英文本 [M]. 北京：中华书局，2000.

[7] 张金明，陆雪春 . 中国古铜镜鉴赏图录 [M]. 北京：中国民族摄影艺术出版社，2002.

[8] 文物精华编辑委员会 . 文物精华 [M]. 北京：文物出版社，1964.

[9] 谭维四 . 湖北出土文物精华 [M]. 武汉：湖北教育出版社，2001.

[10] 常州市博物馆 . 常州文物精华 [M]. 北京：文物出版社，1998.

[11] 镇江博物馆 . 镇江文物精华 [M]. 合肥：黄山书社，1997.

[12] 贵州省文化厅，贵州省博物馆 . 贵州文物精华 [M]. 贵阳：贵州人民出版社，2005.

[13] 徐良玉 . 扬州馆藏文物精华 [M]. 南京：江苏古籍出版社，2001.

[14] 昭陵博物馆，陕西历史博物馆 . 昭陵文物精华 [M]. 西安：陕西人民美术出版社，1991.

[15] 南通博物苑 . 南通博物苑文物精华 [M]. 北京：文物出版社，2005.

[16] 邯郸市文物研究所 . 邯郸文物精华 [M]. 北京：文物出版社，2005.

[17] 张秀生，刘友恒，聂连顺，等 . 中国河北正定文物精华 [M]. 北京：文化艺术出版社，1998.

[18] 陕西省咸阳市文物局 . 咸阳文物精华 [M]. 北京：文物出版社，2002.

[19] 安阳市文物管理局 . 安阳文物精华 [M]. 北京：文物出版社，2004.

[20] 深圳市博物馆 . 深圳市博物馆文物精华 [M]. 北京：文物出版社，1998.

[21]《中国文物精华》编辑委员会 . 中国文物精华（1993）[M]. 北京：文物出版社，1993.

[22] 夏路，刘永生.山西省博物馆馆藏文物精华 [M].太原：山西人民出版社，1999.

[23] 文物精华编辑委员会.文物精华 [M].文物出版社，1957.

[24] 山西博物院，湖北省博物馆.荆楚长歌：九连墩楚墓出土文物精华 [M].太原：山西人民出版社，2011.

[25] 刘广堂，石金鸣，宋建忠.晋国雄风：山西出土两周文物精华 [M].沈阳：万卷出版公司，2009.

[26] 沈君山，王国平，单迎红.滦平博物馆馆藏文物精华 [M].北京：中国文联出版社，2012.

[27] 张家口市博物馆.张家口市博物馆馆藏文物精华 [M].北京：科学出版社，2011.

[28] 浙江省文物考古研究所.浙江考古精华 [M].北京：文物出版社，1999.

[29] 故宫博物院.故宫雕刻珍萃 [M].北京：紫禁城出版社，2004.

[30] 故宫博物院紫禁城出版社.故宫博物院藏宝录 [M].上海：上海文艺出版社，1986.

[31] 首都博物馆.大元三都 [M].北京：科学出版社，2016.

[32] 新疆维吾尔自治区博物馆.新疆出土文物 [M].北京：文物出版社，1975.

[33] 王兴伊，段逸山.新疆出土涉医文书辑校 [M].上海：上海科学技术出版社，2016.

[34] 刘学春.刍议医药卫生文物的概念与分类标准 [J].中华中医药杂志，2016，31（11）:4406-4409.

[35] 上海古籍出版社.中国艺海 [M].上海：上海古籍出版社，1994.

[36] 紫都，岳鑫.一生必知的 200 件国宝 [M].呼和浩特：远方出版社，2005.

[37] 谭维四.湖北出土文物精华 [M].武汉：湖北教育出版社，2001.

[38] 张建青.青海彩陶收藏与鉴赏 [M].北京：中国文史出版社，2007.

[39] 银景琦.仡佬族文物 [M].南宁：广西人民出版社，2014.

[40] 廖果，梁峻，李经纬.东西方医学的反思与前瞻 [M].北京：中医古籍出版社，2002.

[41] 梁峻，张志斌，廖果，等.中华医药文明史集论 [M].北京：中医古籍出版社，2003.

[42] 郑蓉，庄乾竹，刘聪，等.中国医药文化遗产考论 [M].北京：中医古籍出版社，2005.